CLARIFYING CONCEPTS in NURSING RESEARCH

Editor

Audrey G. Gift, PhD, RN, FAAN, is an Associate Professor at the University of Pennsylvania, School of Nursing and Associate Director of the Center for Nursing Research. In addition, she serves as Director of Nursing Research for the University of Pennsylvania Health System. She is best known for her many clinical studies and publications dealing with dyspnea. She has used her intellectual and research skills in developing the concept of dyspnea. She currently serves on the American Thoracic Society's multidisciplinary, international task force to develop a statement on dyspnea. Dr. Gift has been a fellow in the American Academy of Nursing since 1992, served on the Board of the American Nurses Foundation from 1994-1996 and as chair of the American Nurses Association Council for Nursing Research from 1994-1996. She is an editor of the journal *Scholarly Inquiry for Nursing Practice.* In addition, she is Research Editor for *Prospectives in Respiratory Nursing,* and on the Editorial Board of *Heart & Lung.*

Editors of *Scholarly Inquiry for Nursing Practice*

Harriet R. Feldman, Ph.D., R.N., F.A.A.N., Pace University

Ruth Bernstein Hyman, Ph.D., Albert Einstein College of Medicine.

Barbara Kos-Munson, Ph.D., R.N., C.S., Adelphi University.

Audrey Gift, Ph.D., F.A.A.N., University of Pennsylvania

Pierre Woog, Ph.D., Adelphi University

CLARIFYING CONCEPTS in NURSING RESEARCH

Audrey G. Gift, PhD, RN, FAAN, Editor

 Springer Publishing Company

Springer Publishing Company, Inc.
536 Broadway
New York, NY 10012-3955

Cover design by Margaret Dunin
Acquisitions Editor: Ruth Chasek
Production Editor: Matt Fenton

97 98 99 00 01 / 5 4 3 2 1

Library of Congress Cataloging-in-Publication Data

Clarifying concepts in nursing research / [edited by] Audrey G. Gift.
    p. cm.
    Articles drawn from Scholarly inquiry for nursing practice, v. 10, no. 3, 1996.
    Includes bibliographical references and index.
    ISBN 0-8261-9980-1
    1. Nursing models.   2. Concepts.   I. Gift, Audrey G. II.
    Scholarly inquiry for nursing practice.
        [DNLM: 1. Nursing Research. 2. Concept Formation.
        3. Models, Nursing. WY 20.5 C591 1997]
RT84.5.C56 1997
610.73'072—dc21
DNLM/DLC
for Library of Congress   97-9521
                                               CIP

Contents

Contributors

Maritza Cerdas Tasón, PhD
Research Associate
Pennsylvania State University
School of Nursing
University Park, PA

Carol Estwing Ferrans, PhD, RN, FAAN
Assistant Professor
University of Illinois at Chicago
School of Nursing
Chicago, IL

DeAnne K. Hilfinger Messias, RN, MS
University of California at San Francisco
School of Nursing
San Francisco, CA

Judith E. Hupcey, RN, EdD
Pennsylvania State University
School of Nursing
University Park, PA

Harriet Kitzman, PhD, RN
Associate Professor of Nursing
School of Nursing
Associate Professor of Pediatrics
School of Medicine and Dentistry
University of Rochester
Rochester, NY

Elizabeth R. Lenz, PhD, RN, FAAN
Associate Dean of Research
  and Doctoral Studies
Columbia University
School of Nursing
New York, NY

Renee Milligan, PhD, RN
Assistant Professor
Georgetown University
School of Nursing
Washington, DC

Carl Mitcham, PhD
Associate Professor of Philosophy
Director of Science Technology
  and Society Program
Pennsylvania State University
College of Engineering
University Park, PA

Janice M. Morse, PhD, FAAN
Professor
Pennsylvania State University
School of Nursing
University Park, PA

Peggy L. Parks, PhD
Professor
University of Maryland
School of Nursing
Baltimore, MD

Linda C. Pugh, PhD, RNC
Director, Center for Nursing Research
Hershey Medical Center
Hershey, PA

Cathy H. Rosenthal-Dichter, RN, MN, CCRN, FCCM
University of Pennsylvania
School of Nursing
Philadelphia, PA

Introduction

Audrey G. Gift, PhD, RN, FAAN

Concept development is integral to the understanding of nursing practice. It is through the delineation of the phenomena with which nursing is concerned that a language is formulated to facilitate the communication of nursing practice. Locke (1690) stated that labeling abstract ideas enables us to consider phenomena and engage in discourse on them in a way that enhances communication. The labeling of ideas advances science through the communication of knowledge in a more efficient manner than would be possible without such representations. Labeling ideas with words fosters the advancement of nursing science but the process for accomplishing this has not always been clear.

Concept development in nursing has been based in large part on the writings of Wilson (1963) with modifications by nurse authors such as Walker and Avant (1995). The processes they recommend have been designed to accomplish that which Locke proposed, the representation of ideas with words. It clarifies the language used in nursing to ensure that individuals using the same word are clear about its meaning. But nursing is more than ideas; it is a practice profession. Consequently ideas should be relevant to practice. Thus, concept development must be more than labeling ideas with words. The ideas must be tested in the world of nursing practice and involve patients. It is only after they have been validated in the clinical setting that concepts can be embraced in nursing.

This book, which grew out of a special issue of *Scholarly Inquiry for Nursing Practice,* presents critiques of nursing science designed to critically examine past concept development in nursing and to make recommendations for the future. In addition, examples of concept development are provided that follow the recommendations available up to this point, those based on Wilsonian tradition, as well as those that demonstrate how concept development might proceed in the future. The authors, however, do not all use the same term to describe this process. Concept development is the term used most often to encompass the entire conceptual process. It can include techniques such as concept analysis, concept synthesis, and concept derivation (Walker & Avant, 1995) or defining, differentiating, delineating antecedents and consequences, modeling, analogizing, and synthesizing (Meleis, 1991). Others, however, prefer the original language of Wilson, who used the term concept analysis to describe the process by which phenomena of interest are defined and delineated. It is hoped this difference in terminology will not be distracting to the reader.

In the first chapter "Concept Analysis in Nursing: A Critique of Wilsonian Methods" by Hupcey, Morse, Lenz, & Tasón, current models used for concept analysis in nursing are explored and critiqued. These authors focus on that which has been written to date about concept analysis, which involves the development of a concept from the available literature (Walker & Avant, 1995). Comparing and contrasting the writings presently used as guides for concept analysis helps to evaluate the steps in the process and to determine which are essential for nursing science. The authors evaluate the state of nursing science in light of the processes outlined for the delineation of concepts. They focus on Wilson's original writings which have been the "gold standard" for concept development in nursing to this point.

The two chapters that follow are examples that follow the Wilsonian guidelines for concept development. They are exemplars of how this technique can be used in the beginning stages of concept development when concept clarity is vital. The chapter by Rosenthal-Dichter, "The Pediatric Physiologic Stress Response: A Concept Analysis," adheres to Walker and Avant's guidelines for concept development. Rosenthal demonstrates that the techniques recommended for concept development can be used to delineate the physiological concept of stress response in a pediatric population. A physiological concept was included because it is important to apply a similar level of scientific rigor to these concepts as is applied to psychosocial phenomena. Physiological concepts may have multiple meanings in a manner similar to psychosocial phenomena. For example, a study of stress in which stress is defined in terms of the stressor, such as number and severity of life changes, would lead to a different research study than would be suggested for a study of stress focusing on the stress response. Rosenthal-Dichter develops the concept of the stress response for the pediatric population. Much has been written about this topic but little is specific to the pediatric population. She developed her concept by using actual, not fabricated, cases of the stress response.

The chapter by Messias, "Exploring the Concepts of Undocumentedness: The Meaning of a Person's Immigration Status to Nursing Care," demonstrates concept development at an even earlier stage than the previous chapter. The process of concept exploration is not specifically described by Wilson, but is in that tradition. It involves forming a conceptual and contextualized operational definition, identifying characteristics, and drawing the relationship of the concept to nursing and health. An analysis of the social, cultural, historic, economic, political, and legislative contexts of the concept are also a part of concept exploration and are especially important for undocumentedness which can only be understood in light of these contexts. This chapter is an example of concept analysis for a concept new to nursing.

The chapter by Morse, Hupcey, Mitchem, and Lenz, "Choosing a Strategy for Concept Analysis in Nursing Research: Moving Beyond Wilson," is meant to set the stage for concept development that goes beyond what has commonly been written on the topic. The authors contend that a variety of techniques are needed in nursing for concept development. Different techniques are to be used for different stages of concept development. For instance, qualitative techniques are appropriate to develop a new concept and to examine its boundaries with other concepts. In contrast, a critical analysis of the literature requires that a sufficient amount already be written about the concept to allow for analysis. Quantitative methods, such as those used to develop a measurement instrument, are appropriate when fine-tuning a concept. Factor analysis can be used to establish the construct validity or dimensionality of the concept. Implied, but not explicit, in their discussion is the expectation that as one develops a program of research and refines a concept, various techniques will be used at different stages.

The two chapters that follow are examples of concepts that have evolved within a program of research extending 10 or more years and often in collaboration with others. The researchers have used a variety of techniques to fully develop their concept and define its boundaries. Milligan, Lenz, Parks, Pugh and Kitzman, in their chapter "Postpartum Fatigue: Clarifying a Concept," describe the variety of methods they used to delineate and differentiate postpartum fatigue within a program of research. The first step was to examine the literature to develop the initial definition. This was similar to the beginning steps of concept analysis as recommended by Walker and Avant (1995). The notion of postpartum fatigue was expanded with the use of qualitative methods that allowed it to be differentiated from postpartum depression. The words of the new mothers served as the empirical basis for further development of the concept and exploration of its boundaries.

Milligan and colleagues then progressed in their concept development by using quantitative methods to delineate the dimensions of the concept and to demonstrate that fatigue had physical and mental components. They also used quantitative methods to determine the antecedents and effects of postpartum fatigue. The expansion beyond the concept itself to those phenomena that precede or are affected by it resembles theory building. This leads one to wonder where it is that concept development ends and middle-range theory building begins. Using Suppe's (1993) description of middle-range theories as containing measurable concepts bound by postulated relationships, these authors are clearly on the road to theory building. Thus, this chapter also emphasizes the dynamic nature of concept development and theory building (Lenz et al., 1995). Concepts are not defined and then set in stone forever;

rather, they evolve and change over time as new knowledge is brought forth within a program of research.

The last chapter, "Development of a Conceptual Model of Quality of Life," describes Ferrans's development of the concept of quality of life. The initial intent of this author's work was to operationalize the concept in a way that would lead to the development of an instrument to measure quality of life. The desire was to produce an outcome measure for research. Using the self-report of patients, qualitative methods were employed to develop the initial thinking about the concept. Later, quantitative methods were used to validate the findings derived from the qualitative methods. Thus, this concept was developed initially using an empirical approach rather than a search of the literature. This is a somewhat different way to develop a new or emerging concept than that used by others and emphasizes the need for nursing to have a variety of techniques to use for concept development. The most appropriate method depends on the nature of the concept and the knowledge available related to the concept at the time. When Ferrans began her work there was much written about quality of life but there was no agreed upon definition. She chose to develop her ideas from the opinions of patients. Adding to the richness of this work is the validation of the concept of quality of life cross-culturally.

Comparing and contrasting concepts across cultures gives the concepts further validation in much the same way as standardized tools are validated. Ferrans emphasizes the importance of validating concepts with individuals who are exclusively within the culture rather than bilingual individuals who may share ideas and values from both cultures. Cross-cultural validation is rarely mentioned as a step in concept development but should be given more attention in our ever diversifying world.

Concept development in nursing had its beginnings from the writings of Wilson and those who adapted Wilson's ideas to nursing. Their recommendations make a valuable contribution to the essential beginning steps in concept development by serving as a guide to the clarification of ideas. But concept development does not end with the completion of a single study. Those who develop a program of research test their initial ideas about a concept with their research. This sustained effort of nurse researchers and the constant testing of ideas using qualitative and/or quantitative methodologies facilitates the refinement of ideas. It may be only after the development of the wisdom that 10 or more years of research in an area brings that important insights are revealed. This is typical of the social sciences, in which the most valuable contributions have been made by those more established in their careers.

In nursing we have examined the writings of our scholars expecting consistency in their thoughts over time. But that does not appear to be the model practiced or desired by other social science disciplines. It has also not been the practice of those nurses who maintain a sustained program of research. In nursing research such as that of Merle Mishel with her model of uncertainty (Mishel, 1981, 1990), Milligan and Ferrans who describe their work in this book, as well as my own program of research with dyspnea (Gift, 1991; Gift, Plaut, & Jacox, 1986; Gift & Pugh, 1991; Lenz et al., 1997), the concept has changed and expanded over time. Our work demonstrates the dynamic nature of the social sciences and the importance of a sustained effort in a program of research over many years to bring forth significant scientific insights in nursing. In a program of research a concept can evolve from simply meeting the epistemological principle of being clearly defined and well differentiated from other concepts to that of meeting the pragmatic principle of being applicable to the world. As the concept matures even further, the antecedents and consequences of the concept are demonstrated and it evolves into a framework that sets the stage for the building of middle-range theory. The logical principle of being systematically related to other concepts is then explicated. These principles have been defined by Morse, Hupcey, Mitcham, and Lenz (1996). This book serves as a guide to the evolving and dynamic nature of concept development that is essential to a sustained program of nursing research that enhances conceptual clarity and leads to the building of middle-range theory.

REFERENCES

Gift, A. G., Plaut, S. M., & Jacox, A. K. (1986). Psychologic and physiologic factors related to dyspnea in subjects with chronic obstructive pulmonary disease. *Heart and Lung, 15,* 595-601.

Gift, A. G. (1991). Psychologic and physiologic aspects of acute dyspnea in asthmatics. *Nursing Research, 40,* 196-199.

Gift, A. G., & Pugh, L. C. (1993). Dyspnea/fatigue. *Nursing Clinics of North America, 28*(2), 373-384.

Lenz, E., Pugh, L. Gift, A., Milligan, R., & Suppe, F. (1997). The middle-range theory of unpleasant symptoms: An update. *Advances in Nursing Science, 19*(3), 14-26.

Lenz, E., Suppe, F., Gift, A., Pugh, L., & Milligan, R. (1995). Collaborative development of middle-range nursing theories: Toward a theory of unpleasant symptoms. *Advances in Nursing Science, 17*(3), 1-13.

Locke, J. (1690). Essay on human understanding: Book III.

Meleis, A. I. (1991). *Theoretical nursing: Development and progress* (2nd ed.). Philadelphia: J.B. Lippincott.

Mishel, M. H. (1981). The measurement of uncertainty in illness. *Nursing Research, 30,* 258-263.

Mishel, M. H. (1990) Reconceptualization of the uncertainty in illness theory. *Image: Journal of Nursing Scholarship, 22,* 256-262.

Morse, J. M., Hupcey, J. E., Mitcham, C., & Lenz, E. R. (1996). Concept analysis in nursing research: A critical appraisal. *Scholarly Inquiry for Nursing Practice, 10,* 253-277.

Suppe, F. (November 15, 1993) Middle range theories: What they are and why nursing science needs them. Paper presented at the American Nurses Association/Council of Nurse Researchers Symposium, Washington, DC.

Walker, L. O., & Avant, K. C. (1995). *Strategies for theory construction in nursing* (3rd ed.) Norwalk, CT: Appleton & Lange.

Wilson, J. (1963). *Thinking with concepts.* Cambridge University Press: Cambridge.

Part I

Traditional Methods

1

Methods of Concept Analysis in Nursing: A Critique of Wilsonian Methods

Judith E. Hupcey, RN, EdD
Janice M. Morse, PhD (Nurs.),
PhD (Anthro.), FAAN
Elizabeth R. Lenz, PhD, RN, FAAN
Maritza Cerdas Tasón, PhD

...the use of concepts from adjunctive disciplines places a special burden upon theorists and nurses who study theory. It is urgent that the concepts adopted for nursing are accurately reproduced. (Levine, 1995, p.13)

Nurse researchers are paying increasing attention to concepts important to the theoretical foundation of nursing. Since the conceptual basis of nursing theory and research was constructed in a relatively short time using concepts adopted from other disciplines, reexamination of these concepts for relevance and fit is both critical and overdue. In the process of applying borrowed concepts to the nursing context, their definitions were possibly altered, so that reexploration of the meaning, application, and the appropriateness of the borrowed concepts is necessary. Thus, nursing's introspective reevaluation of the discipline's theoretical base is important and urgent.

Despite increased emphasis on concept analysis and the rapidly increasing number of publications exploring concepts, progress has been disconcertingly slow. There has been a disproportionately small gain in knowledge acquisition for the numbers of researchers involved and the numbers of articles published.

Acknowledgments. We thank Carl Mitcham, PhD, for insights and discussions concerning this article. The assistance of Susan Dolan, BA, in the preparation of this manuscript is acknowledged. This research was supported by NIH, NINR, 2R01 NR02130-07 (Morse) and AHCPR, F32 H500094-02 (Hupcey).

In this chapter, we argue that this is an adequate rationale for examining the methods used for concept analysis. We first discuss Wilson's (1963/1969) method of concept analysis and Wilson-derived methods (i.e., those adapted into nursing by Walker and Avant (1983, 1988, 1995) and Chinn and Kramer [Jacobs][1] (1983, 1987, 1991) and further modified by Schwartz-Barcott and Kim (1986, 1993) and Rodgers (1989a, 1993). Excluded from this analysis are concrete physiological phenomena that are also treated as concepts in nursing. Rather, we are primarily interested in more abstract behavioral concepts and the methods used to delineate and clarify them.

In order to achieve these aims, we first described the method proposed by Wilson and then reviewed four Wilson-derived methods of concept analysis used in nursing (see Figure 1.1). Next, chapters that analyzed concepts using these methods were identified, and the application, adherence to the method, and the analytic outcome(s) described in these chapters were critiqued.

A REVIEW OF MAJOR METHODS OF CONCEPT ANALYSIS

Wilson's Method

In the 1960s, Wilson (1963/1969) published a detailed approach to concept analysis, describing 11 techniques (pp. 23-29) intended to guide analysis. It was not Wilson's intent that all techniques be used in all cases; rather, use of a given technique depended on its appropriateness to the question. Wilson's seven "steps" (pp. 94-95) incorporating these 11 techniques are as follows:

(1) Isolate the conceptual question from other questions:
Isolate questions of concept. Conceptual analysis should not be performed on questions of fact, value, or relationships. If research questions contain more than one concept, the individual concepts should be isolated and addressed first.
Develop 'right answers.' As concepts may have multiple meanings and multiple contexts, the researcher must identify the *primary* statement and uses that are at the "heart" of the concept.
(2) Apply the following techniques:
Model cases: Construction of cases or instances, from everyday experiences, that best reflect or illustrate the concept.
Contrary cases: Construction of cases or instances that definitely do not reflect the concept.
Related cases: Construction of cases illustrating instances related to or importantly connected to the concept in some way.

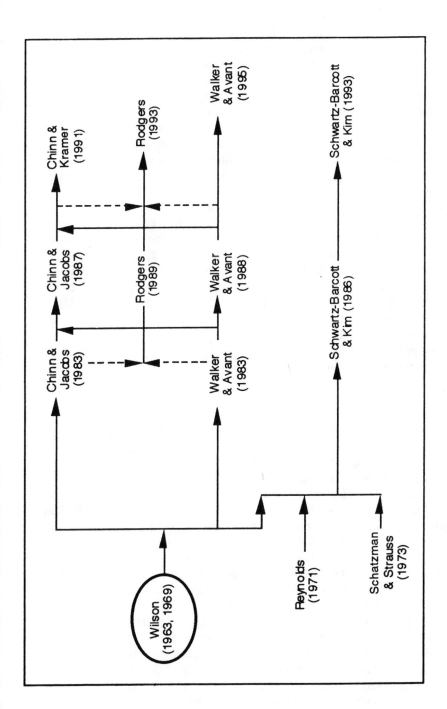

FIGURE 1.1 The evolution of Wilsonian methods of concept analysis.

Borderline cases: Construction of cases that may possibly be an instance of the concept, but the analyst is unsure. Some of the features may be present, but other important features may be missing.

Invented cases: If ordinary experiences do not provide enough instances of the concept to clarify it, imaginary or fabricated cases may be developed to illustrate all the essential features of the concept.

Social context: Explore the nature or circumstance (i.e., context) surrounding the use of the concept, including the "who," "why," and "when."

Underlying anxiety: Investigate the emotive context underlying the concept.

Practical results: Test the practical significance of a concept by creating questions of the concept that have a definitive yes/no answer. This may reveal that the concept, its underlying concepts, or the converse of the concept, is the primary concept of interest or the practical concern.

Results in language: Choose the meaning of the concept that best represents the most useful meaning or delineation of the concept, so that the results are most useful, and "use the word to its fullest advantage" (p. 37).

(3) Conduct an internal dialogue about the concept to question the choices made about the different meanings. If necessary, invent additional cases, moving back and forth until a "basic outline of the concept" (p. 94) is developed. This internal dialogue is the most significant part of the process.

(4) Reanalyze the conceptual question for relevancy.

(5) Compare results of the internal dialogue with the conceptual question and list of points and conclusions to be made.

(6) Write the essay.

(7) Edit the essay.

The major strengths of Wilson's method are the following: (1) The isolation of concepts occurs by first examining a situation or a passage from literature or scientific writings and then choosing the important concept that will be analyzed; (2) Although the cases are "constructed," they are constructed from actual or everyday situations which not only use the concept, but are relevant to the analysis; (3) Invented cases are only constructed when sufficient numbers of actual cases are not available to adequately illustrate the concept; (4) The conceptual features (attributes or characteristics) emerge from the cases, and importantly; (5) The intellectual rigor requisite in concept development is described. The "internal dialogue" and "reanalysis" are listed as distinct processes in the procedure, and the process of analysis continues until adequate results are procured.

It is important to note that it was not Wilson's intent to simplify and clarify methods of concept analysis *per se*, but rather to present methodological guidelines for high school students so that they might acquire the cognitive and writing skills for analyzing concepts. Wilson[2] designed these techniques to be used as class exercises, not as a research method. Despite this, his work has been extremely influential in nursing and forms the basis of concept develop-

ment methods as described by Walker and Avant (1983, 1988, 1995), Chinn
and Kramer [Jacobs], (1983, 1987, 1991), Schwartz-Barcott and Kim (1986,
1993), and Rodgers (1989a, 1993) (see Figure 1.1). Each of these methods as
described by these authors will now be summarized with the methodological
steps listed in Table 1.1 and the major contrasting features in Table 1.2.

Walker and Avant

Walker and Avant (1995) described the need for concept development as a
critical component in the development of nursing theory. They have suggested
three types of concept development: concept analysis, concept derivation, and
concept synthesis. The choice of the type of concept development used
depends upon the maturity of the chosen concept. In terms of concept analysis,
they stated that it is done "to distinguish between the defining attributes of a
concept and its irrelevant attributes" and to "...determine the likeness and
unlikeness between concepts" (p. 38). They view the outcome of concept
analysis as tentative because concepts will change over time.

In 1983, Walker and Avant were among the first to bring Wilson's (1963/
1969) techniques of concept analysis into nursing, and these authors' interpretation of Wilson has been most frequently cited in the nursing literature.
Walker and Avant (1983, 1988, 1995) modified Wilson's (1963/1969) 11
techniques into 8 steps for concept analysis, removing the steps related to the
"internal dialogue" and "re-analysis" (see Table 1.1). Though Walker and
Avant (1995) stated that their steps are iterative and that concept analysis "...is
a vigorous intellectual exercise" (p. 47), these integral processes are not clear
in their steps nor in the discussion of how they are implemented.

Walker and Avant (1995) stated that their method is a simplified version of
Wilson which they feel is easy to understand and therefore fairly simple for
beginners to use. For example, Walker and Avant (1983, 1988, 1995) simplified Wilson's first step of *isolate a concept* to *select a concept*. The former
process is far more complex, requiring consideration of *the* appropriate
concept, its boundaries and criteria for delineation (see Table 1.2). Walker and
Avant's technique involves constructing cases just as Wilson recommended;
however, Wilson's cases are constructed from situations which are relevant to
the context of the concept, and from these cases the features associated with
the concept are developed. Walker and Avant, on the other hand, stated that
cases are constructed so that they will include all the previously identified
attributes. Little stress is placed on the construction of cases that are relevant
to nursing context versus a fabricated case just illustrating the concept.

Chinn and Kramer [Jacobs]

Chinn and Jacobs (1987) stated that concept analysis is "...the most fundamental and important process in developing and refining theory" (p. 87). As

TABLE 1.1 Wilsonian Methods: A Comparison of the Steps of the Major Methods

Steps	Wilson (1963/1969)	Walker & Avant (1995)	Chinn & Kramer (1991)	Rodgers (1993) *Evolutionary Method*	Schwartz-Barcott & Kim (1993) *Hybrid Model*
Selecting the concept		1. "Select a concept" (p. 39)	1. Selecting concept (p. 83)	1. "Identify concept of interest & associated expressions" (p. 78)	Theoretical Phase 1. Select a concept (p. 109)
Determining aims and purposes of analysis		2. "Determine aims or purpose of analysis" (p. 39)	2. Clarifying the purpose (p. 84)		
Delineating domain/ boundaries of the concept	1. Isolate questions of the concept and develop right answers (p. 23–24) 2. Apply techniques: • Construct cases • Explore social context • Investigate underlying anxiety	3. "Identify all uses of the concept as possible" (p. 39)	3. Data sources: Examine existing definitions (p. 84) Literature People sources (p. 88–89)	2. Identify and select an appropriate data realm for data collection (p. 78) 3. "Collect data regarding the attributes along with surrogate terms, references, antecedents, & consequences" (p. 78)	2. Search the literature (p. 109)

(Continued)

TABLE 1.1 (Continued)

Steps	Wilson (1963/1969)	Walker & Avant (1995)	Chinn & Kramer (1991)	Rodgers (1993) Evolutionary Method	Schwartz-Barcott & Kim (1993) Hybrid Model
	• Test practical significance • Identify the meaning that best represents the concept			4. "Identify concepts related to the concept of interest" (p. 78)	
Defining internal components and attributes	3. Conduct an internal dialogue (p. 94)	4. "Determine defining attributes" (p. 39)		5. "Analyze data regarding the above characteristics of the concept" (p. 78) 6. "Conduct interdisciplinary or temporal comparisons, or both, if desired" (p. 78)	3. Deal with meaning and measurement (p. 109) 4. Choose a working definition (p. 109)
Developing prototypes	Construct cases: model, borderline, related, contrary, and invented (p. 28–32) 4. Reanalyze questions for relevancy (p. 94)	5. "Construct a model case" (p. 39) 6. "Construct borderline, related, contrary, invented, and illegitimate cases" (p. 39)	Construct cases: model, contrary, related, borderline (p. 85–87) 4. Explore contexts and values (p. 89)	7. "Identify a model case of the concept, if appropriate" (p. 78)	Fieldwork Phase 1. Set the stage 2. Negotiate entry 3. Select cases 4. Collect and analyze data (p. 109)

(Continued)

TABLE 1.1 (Continued)

Steps	Wilson (1963/1969)	Walker & Avant (1995)	Chinn & Kramer (1991)	Rodgers (1993) Evolutionary Method	Schwartz-Barcott & Kim (1993) Hybrid Model
Determining developmental outcomes	Explore social context • Investigate underlying anxiety • Test practical significance • Identify the meaning that best represents the concept (p. 94)	7. "Identify antecedents and consequences" (p. 39)		[Incorporated into data collection]	
Identifying indices	5. Compare result of self-dialogue with questions and conclusions 6. Write the essay (p. 95) 7. Edit the essay (p. 95)	8. "Define empirical referents" (p. 39)	5. Formulate criteria (p. 90)	8. "Identify hypotheses and implications for further development" (p. 78)	Analytic Phase "Weighing, working, and writing up the findings" (p. 109)

TABLE 1.2 Comparisons of Purpose and Descriptions of Wilsonian Methods of Concept Development

Principles	Wilson (1969)	Walker & Avant (1995)	Chinn & Kramer (1991)	Rodgers (1993)	Schwartz-Barcott & Kim (1993)
Selection of concept	Isolate the important concept from literary or scientific passages	According to interest (p. 40)	According to idea of interest (p. 83)	According to interest (p. 78)	From an encounter in a real-life nursing situation (p. 110)
Aims and purpose of analysis	To teach high school students to think purposively (pp. x–ix)	To clarify meaning; Develop operational definitions; Add to theory (p. 40)	To create conceptual meaning for theory building (p. 79)	To add new knowledge (p. 75)	To develop theory for nursing practice (p. 108)
Data source	Identify the *primary* statement that best represents the concept (p. 27)	"...may use dictionary, thesauruses, colleagues, and available literature" Include all uses of the concept (p. 40–41)	Dictionary, cases, pictures, music, literature, people (p. 84, 88–89)	Rigorous and systematic sampling of multi-disciplinary literature (p. 90)	Broad systematic multi-disciplinary review of literature (p. 112)

(Continued)

TABLE 1.2 (Continued)

Principles	Wilson (1969)	Walker & Avant (1995)	Chinn & Kramer (1991)	Rodgers (1993)	Schwartz-Barcott & Kim (1993)
Process/ procedure	Work "back and forth" between cases and the statements (p. 94) Constructs cases to identify the features (p. 28–32) Explore usage, circumstances, emotive context application, and lexical definition Conduct internal dialogue and reanalysis of question (p. 94)	List characteristics that occur over and over during your review (p. 41) Construct cases to include all attributes (p. 42–45) Identify prior events and results of the occurrence of the concept (p. 45)	Construct cases; identify tentative criteria for the concept (p. 85–87) Examine cases in terms of social contexts, and values to help clarify the meaning (pp. 89–90)	Conduct content/ thematic analysis (p. 85–86) Identify a universal model case (p. 87)	Consider all definitions and develop a working (nursing) definition (p. 113) Conduct field-work and analyze data May develop cases (p. 113–123)
Outcome	Relevant comparison of points and conclusion (p. 94). Essay (p. 95)	Locating classes of actual phenomena that demonstrate existence of concept (p. 46)	Criteria that amplify the meaning of the concept and "suggest direction for theory development" (p. 90)	Plan for further investigation by identifying hypotheses etc. (p. 87–89)	Interface theoretical and empirical observations and evaluate importance for nursing (p. 124–125)

they saw it the purpose of analyzing a concept in relation to the development of theory "is to identify, clarify, and examine the word label, the phenomenon represented by the label, and the values, feeling, and attitudes that are associated with both the symbol and the phenomenon" (p. 88). The outcomes of concept analysis are also described by Chinn and Jacobs (1987) as tentative, since the definition of the concept and the criteria associated with its presence in a particular context "are subject to alteration and change as new evidence becomes available" (p. 90).

Chinn and Kramer [Jacobs] first delineated their method of concept analysis in 1983, also attributing their method to Wilson (1963/1969) (see Figure 1.1). As shown in Table 1.1, Chinn and Kramer's (1991) steps differ from Walker and Avant's method by omitting the step, *identifying antecedents and consequences*, and by *formulating criteria* (i.e., Walker and Avant's step *delineate defining attributes*), once all the data have been collected and analyzed and the values and social context taken into account. Later (1991), they also placed cases under the category of "data sources" and included numerous potential sources of data that may also be used during the analysis (see Table 1.2).

Chinn and Kramer's method of concept development appears closer to Wilson than Walker and Avant's explication of Wilson. They follow Wilson by constructing cases to identify features associated with the concept and differentiating those features (criteria) that are truly related to the concept of interest and those that are not. They also examine the social context of the cases, as well as the values associated with the concept, as does Wilson. It is not until all of these areas are examined that Chinn and Kramer expect criteria to be formulated. Though Chinn and Kramer described examining many areas in the process of concept analysis, they also did not stress the requisite intellectual rigor that Wilson describes.

Schwartz-Barcott and Kim

The *hybrid model* of concept analysis was developed as a result of a perceived lack of an adequate approach to concept development for the process of theory building. Schwartz-Barcott and Kim (1993) stated that they developed a method "that would help to ensure that —

1. The concepts selected for analysis would be integral to nursing practice.
2. The literature reviewed would be broad enough to capture the commonalties and extremes in conceptualization and usage of the concept across disciplines.
3. The focus of analysis would be on the essential aspects of definition and measurement.
4. Analysis from the literature would be tightly integrated with the empirical aspects of the definition and measurement" (p. 108).

The *hybrid model* combines Wilson's (1963/1969) analytic approach for case selection and analysis with Reynolds's (1971) analytic approach for data collection and analysis, and Schatzman and Strauss's (1973) field work techniques (see Figure 1.1). There are some aspects of this model that have Wilsonian underpinnings, yet the overall approach (the combination of the three phases: theoretical, fieldwork, and analytical) is quite different (see Table 1.1). The main similarities with Wilson (1963/1969) are in the selection of the concept. Though Schwartz-Barcott and Kim (1993) use a real (nursing) situation to identify a concept, and Wilson's students use book passages, both approaches carefully examine the context and thoughtfully identify the concept to be analyzed. Wilson's influence is also seen during case selection when model, contrary, borderline, and related cases may be developed if the concept remains unclear. An important difference with the *hybrid model* is that the cases are identified from empirical data and not constructed by the researcher. The final important link between this model and Wilson is the active movement back and forth between the phases and re-analysis of the data until the concept is clearly understood (see Table 1.2).

Rodgers

Rodgers (1989a, 1993) stated that she developed an *evolutionary method* of concept analysis using the philosophical literature as its basis. This method emphasizes conceptual change, indicating "that concept development must be an ongoing process, with no realistic end point... Attempts to delineate clear boundaries, to distinguish a concept from its context, or to view it apart from a network of related concepts, as is often done with concept analysis, are not consistent with this view" (p. 77). The actual purpose of undertaking concept analysis appears to be the development of knowledge.

Rodgers stated that the method is consistent with the philosophical underpinnings and "resembles the approaches presented by Wilson (1963) and popularized in nursing by Walker and Avant (1983, 1988) and Chinn and Jacobs (1987) Chinn and Kramer (1991)" (Rodgers, 1993, p. 77). As seen in Table 1.1, the procedures are similar to those presented by Walker and Avant (1995); however, the ordering of the steps is somewhat different. Consistent with Wilson and Chinn and Kramer, Rodgers identifies (not constructs) her "model case" after the data are analyzed; however, the attributes, surrogate terms, antecedents, and consequences are compiled during the process of data collection. A step involving interdisciplinary or temporal comparison (see Wilson, 1963/1969), may be included, but Rodgers does not mention this process during the discussion of the implementation of her method. There are three main differences associated with Rodgers's *evolutionary method* (see Table 1.2). First, "emphasis is placed especially on the conduct of a rigorous and systematic study. Specific considerations have been noted in regard to sample selection or literature review" (Rodgers, 1993, p. 90). Rodgers clearly stresses this aspect in her discussion of the use of her method. Second, Rodgers uses a qualitative approach to data analysis. Finally, Rodgers differentiates her method by not emphasizing the development of cases but the identification of concepts that are related to the concept being analyzed. Though in reality this step is similar to the development of related cases, since the cases include related concepts, Rodgers (1993) states: "related cases are limited to a focus on application of the specific concept of interest, or situations that demonstrate perhaps some, but not all, of the attributes of the concept being analyzed...it does not provide any insight into what *other* concepts might be relevant in similar situations" (p.84).

ASSESSMENT OF WILSON-DERIVED METHODS

In this section, the major methods of concept analysis derived from Wilson will be critiqued, and the major processes in the methods will be compared. The strengths as well as the weaknesses will also be described.

Walker and Avant

Walker and Avant made an important contribution by introducing procedures for concept development into nursing, and these procedures were immediately incorporated as a standard component of theory courses. The procedure for concept analysis was clearly explicated in a way that could be readily taught and easily used by the students. This has become a "mixed blessing," however, as the task of concept development is one of the most crucial for the development of nursing theory and research, and designating this responsibility to doctoral students with limited experience and time, as with the development of theory, "makes light of nursing as a serious intellectual inquiry" (Stevens, 1984, p. ix).

There are serious limitations to the concept development procedures as they were changed in the process of adaptation. Whereas Wilson obtained his definitions from his cases, Walker and Avant construct cases that fit attributes derived from the dictionary and other definitions. They use limited sources of data, and provide no rationale for incorporating all dictionary definitions, even those that are irrelevant (e.g., coping=coping saw). Because there is limited case development—only one case per category—and these cases have been constructed to fit the attributes, they serve as deductively derived examples to illustrate the predetermined attributes rather than serving as the basis for inductively identifying attributes. This reverse procedure is the major threat to the method's validity.

Another serious concern is that despite the fact that Walker and Avant (1995) stated that attributes may be *identical to the empirical referent* (p. 46), in effect, attributes (Step 4) and empirical referents (Step 8) do not fulfill the same function and are even defined differently by Walker and Avant. Attributes are defined as "characteristics associated with concepts," and empirical referents, as "classes or categories of phenomena that by their existence or presence demonstrate the occurrence of the concept itself" (p. 46).

Most serious is Walker and Avant's failure to communicate the essential intellectual work of concept analysis. Their method does not describe Wilson's "internal dialogue" and the "re-analysis" of the emerging concept. Furthermore, they have omitted the necessity of synthesizing the steps with one another to produce a comprehensive description of the concept in the conclusion.

Chinn and Kramer [Jacobs]

Chinn and Kramer [Jacobs] developed concept analysis with the goal of contributing to theory development. Although their method was first published the same year as Walker and Avant's (1983) and acknowledged Wilson in later editions, Chinn and Kramer gave attribution to Walker and Avant. However, their method is less detailed than Walker and Avant's and this vagueness and lack of detail make their method difficult to follow.

The main strength of their method is that the criteria are developed from the cases, which is consistent with Wilson's approach. Despite the fact that these cases are constructed, they are later tested and looked at through social context and in terms of the values associated with the concept, thus contributing to their validity.

Schwartz-Barcott and Kim

The *hybrid model* of concept development has many aspects that make up for qualities missing from both Walker and Avant and Chinn and Kramer's [Jacobs] methods. This model includes using actual nursing situations as the basis of concept selection, conducting an extensive multidisciplinary literature review, collecting and analyzing empirical data, identifying 'real' cases, and working back and forth between the empirical data and literature. The use of qualitative empirical data and actual cases enriches the analysis possible with the use of this model. The suggestion by the authors that only a limited selection of actual cases need to be observed and then analyzed, however, impairs the rigor, validity, and completeness of concept explication. Though Schwartz-Barcott and Kim say that selecting the cases depends on the concept to be studied, they also say that a large number of cases is unnecessary with this type of research. They do not consider whether the data are truly saturated and therefore actually representative of the concept of interest in its entirety. In addition, the use of limited cases from one nursing situation and the development of a conceptual definition to fit only one nursing situation limit the applicability of the concept to other nursing situations.

Rodgers

Rodgers's method compensates somewhat for the lack of adequacy of data as seen with other Wilson-derived methods by using an inductive approach. She also emphasizes a rigorous and systematic sample selection and data collection process which is lacking in both Walker and Avant's and Chinn and Kramer's [Jacobs] methods (Rodgers stated that her method would fit both the literature as data and empirical data, but her discussion of sample selection is only related to the literature). In terms of her overall approach to concept analysis, Rodgers says that a philosophical foundation was used in the development of the *evolutionary method*; however, this foundation is not reflected in the method itself. Rodgers's (1989a, 1993) method of concept analysis uses qualitative methods in an important attempt to avoid confabulated data and thus improve rigor and validity. Rodgers (1993) seems to undermine her own efforts by recommending delaying analysis of the data until all data have been collected, thus violating standard qualitative procedures. Furthermore, though she asserts that concepts are context bound, and large quantities of qualitative data are collected, Rodgers (1993) recommends presenting a single model case (incident) that is generic enough to *encompass all contexts*. Thus, this step results in the loss of richness otherwise obtained from the synthesis of qualitative data when more orthodox procedures are followed. In addition, selecting an incident that "encompasses all contexts" contradicts her earlier statement that concepts are "context bound" (p. 77). Thus most of the advantages obtained from using actual data are lost with this case study approach.

A final concern with Rodgers's approach relates to her Step 6, *conduct interdisciplinary or temporal comparison, if desired*. This phase of concept development lacks significance because of the statement *if desired*. Emphasizing the lack of importance Rodgers places on this critical part of concept analysis is the fact that this process is ignored during her discussion of the implementation of her method.

Global Limitations of the Wilson-Derived Methods

In summary the limitations found in most of the Wilson-derived methods of concept development are:

1. Incomplete and vague descriptions of the application of the method
2. Lack of clarity about what is a suitable concept for analysis or how you truly choose a concept
3. Lack of discussion about the intellectual rigor (internal dialogue) involved in concept development (most methods do not even have it as a step) and
4. Failure to discuss (with the exception of Schwartz-Barcott and Kim) how the steps are integrated with one another, despite assertions that the process is iterative and not a cookbook or stepwise procedure.

UTILIZATION OF THE METHODS

Walker and Avant

Walker and Avant's explication of Wilson's method has been used most frequently by nurse researchers and by students in nursing doctoral programs. The concepts that have been selected for analysis and published by nurse researchers using Walker and Avant's method are shown in Table 1.3. Though the range of topics analyzed is impressive, Walker and Avant's limited methodological discussion of Step 1, *select a concept*, has apparently led researchers to choose concepts for analysis for reasons that are not always clear. The outcomes resulting from these analyses, even if well done, are, therefore, not always significant to nursing.

Determining the aims or the *purpose of analysis* is the second step identified by Walker and Avant. As shown in Table 1.3, the primary reason for concept analysis stated by nurse researchers using this method was concept clarification, although a few have used Walker and Avant's technique to assist with theory development or to operationalize a concept. Despite the various purposes for concept analysis, there is no apparent variation in Walker and Avant's method by any of these authors.

Identify all uses of the concept, Step 3, is poorly performed by the researchers using this method. Rather than seeking comprehensive definitions from the literature, most authors have been perfunctory in limiting their search to dictionary definitions. Dictionary definitions tend to reflect everyday usage, are not context or discipline bound, and rarely reflect the subtle nuances of their use in nursing or health care.

Since many of the researchers identify limited definitions of the concept in Step 3, Walker and Avant's Step 4, *determining defining attributes*, becomes a trivial exercise with authors simply picking out the key words from the chosen definitions. Of even greater concern, some researchers present attributes that are basically the same as dictionary definitions. For example, in the concept analyses of intuition (Rew, 1986), expert (Jasper, 1994), and crisis (Geissler, 1984), the attributes are very similar to the initial dictionary definitions of the concept. This is a serious limitation, for the attributes play a significant role in the transformation of the concept to a higher level of abstraction. This process of abstraction links the concept to other concepts and provides indicators that may later be operationalized. Thus, the lack of intellectual effort and rigor at this point severely curtails the usefulness of the inquiry.

Due to confusion in the terminology regarding attributes and empirical referents in the methodological discussion by Walker and Avant, some authors have used the *same terms* as both attributes and empirical referents (for example, see Allan's [1993] analysis of feminism), and the lack of consider-

TABLE 1.3 Adherence to Walker and Avant's (1983, 1987) Method

Concept (Author)	1	2	3	4	5	6a	6b	6c	6d	6e	7a	7b	8
Belonging (Hagerty et al., 1992)	x	Instrument development	x	x	x	x	x	x	x	-	x	x	x
Chronic Sorrow (Lindgren et al., 1992)	x	Theory development	x	x	x	x	x	x	x	x	x	x	-
Crisis (Geissler, 1984)	x	Concept clarification	x	x	x	-	x	x	-	-	x	x	?
Decision Making (Matteson & Hawkins, 1990)	x	Concept clarification	x	x	x	x	x	x	x	-	x	x	x
Dignity (Mairis, 1994)		Concept clarification	x	x	x	-	x	x	x	-	x	x	x
Empowerment (Hawks, 1992)	x	Concept clarification	x	x	x	-	x	x	x	-	x	x	?
Expert (Jasper, 1994)	x	Concept clarification	x	x	x	x	x	x	x	x	x	x	x
Feminism (Allan, 1993)	x	Concept clarification	x	x	x	x	x	x	x	-	x	x	x
Friendship (Caroline, 1993)	x	Theory development	x	x	x	x	x	x	x	-	x	x	x
Health (Simmons, 1989)	x	Concept clarification	x	x	x	x	x	x	x	-	-	-	-
Hope (Stephenson, 1991)	x	Concept clarification	x	x	-	-	-	-	-	-	x	x	-
Hopelessness (Campbell, 1987)	x	Operationalize	x	x	x	-	-	x	x	-	x	x	x
Intuition (Rew, 1986)	x	Concept clarification	x	x	x	x	x	x	x	-	x	x	x
Mother-Daughter Identification (Boyd, 1985)	x	Theory development	x	x	x	-	x	x	-	-	x	x	x
Power (Hawks, 1991)	x	Concept clarification	x	x	x	-	x	x	x	-	x	x	x
Quality of Life (Meeberg, 1993)	x	Concept clarification	x	x	x	x	x	x	x	x	x	x	x
Reassurance (Teasdale, 1989)	x	Concept clarification	x	x	x	x	x	x	x	-	-	-	x
Self-Neglect (Reed & Leonard, 1989)	x	Concept clarification	x	x	x	x	x	x	x	x	x	x	x
Self-Nurturing (Nemcek, 1987)	x	Concept clarification	x	x	x	-	x	x	x	-	x	x	x
Serenity (Roberts & Fitzgerald, 1991)	x	Evaluate usefulness	x	x	x	x	x	x	x	-	x	x	x
Spiritual Perspective, Hope, Acceptance (Haase et al., 1992)	x	Simultaneous concept clarification	-	x	-	-	-	-	-	-	-	-	-
Trust (Meize-Grochowski, 1994)	x	Operationalize	x	x	x	x	x	x	-	x	x	x	x

*Steps. 1. Select a concept; 2. Aims of analysis; 3. Identify all uses of the concept; 4. Determine defining attributes; 5. Construct a model case; 6. a. Borderline case b. Related case c. Contrary case d. Invented case e. Illegitimate case; 7. a. Antecedents b. Consequences; 8. Define empirical referents.

Key: x = step included; - = step not included; ? = writing is unclear about this step.

ation of the difference between attributes and empirical referents limits the conceptual development of these components.

While all of the authors using Walker and Avant's (1995) explication have constructed a *model case* (Step 5), the *borderline, related, contrary, invented,* and *illegitimate* cases (Step 6) are not constructed in all instances (see Table 1.3). Most notably, authors omitted the construction of the related, invented, and illegitimate cases. Omitting these cases limits the richness that leads to the development of the conceptualization. Richness is also limited by restricting the cases to one example in each area. These gaps in providing examples and writing case studies that are often thin with meager descriptions even further impoverish the "data base." Constructing cases from the researcher's recollections or confabulating them from the researcher's imagination, rather than using rich and meticulously collected observational or interview data, further limits conceptualization. Examples of various types of fabricated cases illustrating these problems include the following:

a) Model case: **Belonging** (Hagerty, Lynch-Sauer, Patusky, Bouwsema, & Collier, 1992)

A young man, a liberal Democrat, enjoys talking with his neighbors and feels himself to be an important part of the community. His neighbors are all conservative Republicans. They tease the Democrat but affectionately comment that he 'keeps them honest in their views'(p. 174).

b) Related case: **Quality of Life** (Meeberg, 1993)

The artist lays down his paintbrush and looks at his newest masterpiece. He exults, 'This is my best work yet.' He can hardly wait to get it framed so he can display the painting. 'How fulfilling it is to be an artist and to see what I can create with my own hands,' he reflects(p. 35).

c) Invented case: **Empowerment** (Hawks, 1992)

A baby bird is nurtured by its mother for several weeks. The mother bird feeds, comforts and keeps the baby bird safe and warm. When it is time for the baby bird to fly, she nudges him out of the nest. He is frightened, but begins to flap his wings as he often watched his mother do. He notices that he is flying and that his mother is right beside him. Eventually he will be able to fly as gracefully as his mother (p. 618).

These fictitious accounts do not substitute for scholarship. Such examples often appear without a discussion of their significance to the concept analysis, thus confusing instead of helping the reader identify their relevance and contribution to the inquiry. The lack of commentary linking each component of the concept analysis is vexing and creates a void in the presentation.

Limiting analysis to a single model case, or even to five cases (i.e., a model case, borderline case, related case, contrary case, and illegitimate case), restricts the level of abstractness and applicability of the emerging attributes. Alternatively, the characteristics may be so abstract that their particular relevance to the concept that they represent is lost; consequently the analysis loses validity. An example of this is Stephenson's (1991) analysis of hope, where the identified attributes are not specific to hope. The four attributes identified are:

1. The object of hope is meaningful to the person;
2. Hope is a process involving thoughts, feelings, behaviors and relationships;
3. There is an element of anticipation;
4. There is a positive future orientation, which is grounded in the present and linked with the past (p. 1459).

These attributes may represent hope but equally well may represent friendship, fear, love, and hate. It is clear that criteria for evaluation of concept development research and standards for reliability and validity need to be developed.

Step 7 is to identify *the antecedents and consequences*. There is confusion about the ordering of this step with some researchers (Caroline, 1993; Hawks, 1991; Reed & Leonard, 1989; Rew, 1986), identifying these before presenting the model cases, thus limiting themselves to the dictionary definitions for identifying the antecedents and consequences. Others more appropriately identify the antecedents and consequences from the model cases. A similar problem occurs with *defining empirical referents* (Step 8). In addition to the empirical referents being confused with attributes, there appears to be some misunderstanding about what an empirical referent actually is. For example, Jasper (1994) uses the step, *empirical referents*, to describe suggestions for future research.

Often in concept development articles using Walker and Avant's approach there are no summary statements, syntheses, or outcomes of major findings listed. In other instances, the outcomes remarkably resemble the dictionary definition presented at the outset, so that the reader is left in a quandary wondering about the purpose of the exercise and what it contributed. One author, astutely recognizing this problem, concluded that research should be done to develop the concept, and reiterated her initial goal; thus her study clearly did not advance knowledge in any way (Nemcek, 1987). Similarly, some analyses were circular, with authors recognizing the limited contribution of their research. For example, when studying *Dignity*, Mairis (1994) explicitly stated that the purpose was *concept clarification*, yet in her conclusions, the author stated: "This concept clarification is neither fully accurate nor complete" (p. 952). Rew (1986), exploring *Intuition*, expressed dissatisfaction with her study by concluding, "Although clarification of intuition through concept analysis has shed light on this concept, the future of nursing as a science and as a profession could depend on willingness to explore it in greater depth and breadth" (p. 27).

Chinn and Kramer [Jacobs]

Two studies (Timmerman, 1991; Warren, 1993) were identified that used Chinn and Jacobs's 1987 method. The results of these studies suffer from the same limitations as those studies by authors who have used Walker and Avant (1983, 1988), partially because they do not follow all the steps as outlined by Chinn and Jacobs. For example, Timmerman's analysis of intimacy followed all of Chinn and Jacobs's (1987) steps except *testing the cases*; however, the steps that were followed were not appropriately carried through. Timmerman developed a theoretical definition, but it is unclear from her written analysis where the actual definition came from. In addition, instead of *constructing cases*, the author explained other concepts that are felt to be related, borderline and contrary to the concept of intimacy. True cases, as defined by Chinn and Jacobs, were not developed. Warren's (1993) analysis of the concept of social isolation has many of the same problems as Timmerman's study. Warren also excluded the step, *testing cases*, and though many definitions of social isolation were given, there was no true examination of these definitions and no theoretical definition of the concept was developed by the author. The criteria formulated for the concept appear to be developed from Carpenito's (1992, as cited in Warren, 1993) definition of the nursing diagnosis, which was already accepted by nursing. It is unknown how the cases were developed and whether the criteria for the concept were developed from the cases or the cases were constructed from these criteria. As a result, Warren's concept analysis did not add new knowledge to nursing.

Schwartz-Barcott and Kim

Schwartz-Barcott and Kim (1993) stated that the *hybrid model* had been used with over 70 concepts; however, only three published articles were actually identified that used this model. All three studies followed the *hybrid model* as described by Schwartz-Barcott and Kim. Phillips (1991) used the *hybrid model* to analyze the concept of chronic sorrow in mothers with ill or disabled children. She chose only three mothers for the study, however, believing that the concept would be observable in these women. Verhulst and Schwartz-Barcott (1993) also chose only four subjects in their analysis of the concept of withdrawal. They chose three subjects who they felt would be typical of a nursing home population and one subject who was thought to be atypical. Madden (1990) analyzed the concept of therapeutic alliance using the *hybrid model*. Though she observed a variety of patients and chose model cases from these observations for specific analysis, she only observed one nurse's interaction with these patients, again leaving the adequacy of collected data in question. Thus while the *hybrid model* potentially improves upon other Wilson-derived models, the use of only three or four prechosen subjects severely limits the analysis of the concept under study.

Rodgers

Five published articles were found that used Rodgers' *evolutionary method.* All of these studies used the literature as data. Rodgers was the sole author or coauthor of four of the articles, and she followed her method as described. Though apparently large numbers of articles were reportedly reviewed during the process of concept analysis, in three of Rodgers's four articles no data sources were cited either in the text or reference sections. Throughout the articles the only reference to concept usage in the literature reviewed was written as "typically authors" (Westra & Rodgers, 1991, p. 278), "reported by authors" (Rodgers & Cowles, 1991, p. 448) or as just "literature" (Rodgers, 1989b, pp. 698-699). This lack of attribution of the definitions and attributes is a concern. Further, although Rodgers (1993) stated that "the attributes of the concept constitute the *real* definition" (p. 83), these definitions do not stand alone and are meaningless without detailed explanations as to how they relate to the concept of interest or without the antecedents and consequences discussed along with the definition. For example, Rodgers and Cowles (1991) stated that "through this analysis, the concept of grief has been defined as a dynamic process that is highly individualized and strongly influenced by existing norms" (p. 454). This definition could equally apply to numerous concepts; specificity to grief would require including the antecedents and consequences. Attree (1993) attempted to use Rodgers's model to analyze the concept of quality. She failed to follow through with the analysis, however, and reviewed only existing meanings and attributes. The review was summarized by saying that she was unable to propose a definition but that the concept of quality was used in many diverse perspectives.

"Combined" Methods

A few researchers have stated that they combined a variety of methods for concept analysis, yet did not provide evidence of their methodology. Most of the time authors chose one or two steps from someone else's method, but provided no real criteria for their choice nor any rationale for combining methods. In addition, the steps chosen were often used out of context and were frequently used incorrectly. For instance, Watson (1991) used Rodgers's (1989a, 1993) step of *identifying and selecting the appropriate realm for data collection*, then used the dictionary as the "data source." Other authors combined the methods, perhaps as a way to legitimize their concept analyses. For example, Gibson (1991), in her analysis of empowerment, cited criteria from diverse sources such as Norris (1982), Rodgers (1989a), Schwartz-Barcott and Kim (1986), and Walker and Avant (1988) to analyze the concept of empowerment, but did not describe how these combined methods were used. In summary, researchers who have combined methods provided no rationale for selecting and mixing procedures, and sometimes did not comply with the intent of the original method. This further weakened their analyses.

Limitations of Concept Analysis Research

In summary, regardless of attempts to synthesize Wilson's method, the research results of those who have used adaptations of Wilson's method remain similarly deficient and lacking in substance. Articles describing concept analyses appear to lack the intellectual investment or the intellectual work that is inherent in inquiry. Steps in the process of analysis remain isolated from each other and thus do not contribute to the information obtained from the previous step. Thus, using adaptations of Wilson's guidelines as a method seems to produce an outcome that lacks cohesion and does not enlighten one step with another or even the phenomenon itself. At the end of the exercise, the findings are usually not culminated or integrated into a conclusive statement, nor is there a discussion about the results presented. There is frequently no integration that builds upon each step; therefore, at the end of the procedure, the results are left hanging without interpretation or a concluding statement. It is often not possible to determine why the results are valid or even what purpose the exercise served.

DISCUSSION

In nursing, the main methods for exploring abstract concepts have been derived from Wilson (1963/1969). Although researchers have recently attempted to rectify the major limitations of the method by incorporating qualitative data, the results often remain insignificant and without substance. The results of concept analyses using Wilson-derived methods lack comprehensiveness, explanatory power, and are superficial. The research does not elucidate nursing phenomena, nor does it add to nursing knowledge in general.

Despite Wilson's (1963/1969) warning that there are "few, if any, fixed rules" (p. 20) and his concern that "there is also the feeling that questions of concept can be settled much more easily than in fact is the case" (p. 17), Wilson's guidelines for analysis were transformed into rigid instructions for achieving conceptual analysis. With the diffusion of his method into nursing, his guidelines have been rendered meaningless and rote. As a result, nurse researchers have been deceived, thinking that by perfunctorily following instructions they would be assured of a worthwhile analytic product. Paradoxically, the reverse was true. Reynolds (1971) noted "that good ideas in clumsy form generally gain wider acceptance than poor ideas in correct form. . . " (p.3). Perhaps in the case of Wilson-derived methods, the adherence to methodologic concerns over content is at the heart of the problem.

It is significant that the modifications of the Wilson method have not greatly improved the outcome of the research. It is time that nurse researchers investigate new methods for concept development. Rodgers's (1989a, 1993) *evolutionary method* of concept analysis using qualitative methods and Schwartz-Barcott and Kim's (1986, 1993) *hybrid method* are important attempts to move from confabulated data to improved rigor. The use of confabulated or recalled experiences in place of data interferes with the very substance of the developing concepts and places nurse researchers at par with the armchair anthropologists of the 1920s. It is imperative that qualitative analysis of observational and interview data, and at later stages of concept development, a careful interplay between quantitative multivariate analysis and conceptualization, replace the shallow, descriptive, single case study approach that appears in the literature.

Preoccupation with the techniques of concept analysis has eclipsed the importance of substance, i. e., delineating the characteristics of the concept itself and the role it plays in explaining reality. Researchers who set out to conduct concept analysis seem to have forgotten that the concept *per se* is only an abstract image of the phenomenon under study. The ultimate purpose of concept inquiry is to enable the researcher to delineate the phenomenon and transform it to an operationalization of the phenomenon. If the Wilson-derived methods are used in a rote manner, and research using these methods is fractionated and reveals little depth of analysis, then the desired purpose is obfuscated. Researchers have forgotten to ask the questions: Why is the method of use? What do I want to find out? Why do I want to know? And, for what purpose? If these questions had been asked of Wilson's method, researchers would have recognized that it has only limited utility. Had researchers been less concerned with the method as a procedure rather than as a technique for ultimately understanding the phenomenon itself, then perhaps there would have been innovative methodological advances in this area. The modifications used in Wilson-derived methods have for the most part failed to correct the basic limitation of the original Wilson method: that it was not intended as a research procedure. The adherence to simplistic techniques reflects enshrinement of the method over the intellectual effort that necessarily accompanies the process of inquiry.

Given the lack of useful results, why then do nurse researchers continue this line of inquiry? Possible explanations are that it is perceived to be easy to follow, and that it is a way to teach doctoral students critical thinking. It is ironic, however, to note that when the foregoing critique of these methods is taken into consideration, they do not truly teach "critical" thinking. Neither is the goal of producing a publishable article adequate rationale for continuing an unproductive line of inquiry. It is the responsibility of researchers to continually question and seek improved methods of conducting research and the responsibility of clinicians to provide substantive direction for this research.

It is irresponsible of reviewers to approve the status quo without questioning the contribution of each article to nursing science.

While it was not the intention of this chapter to critique the other two main approaches to concept analysis (i.e., critical analysis of the literature and qualitative methodologies), examination of the studies using these alternatives reveals that the results appear to be more comprehensive and useful to nursing (see chapter 4). The development of appropriate *techniques* for concept analysis and continued inquiry into the conceptual basis of nursing are the primary tasks for nursing in the 21st century.

NOTES

[1] Kramer, formerly Jacobs.
[2] While Wilson does not cite Wittgenstein, it is probable that his book is an interpretation of Wittgenstein's work.

REFERENCES

Allan, H. T. (1993). Feminism: A concept analysis. *Journal of Advanced Nursing, 18,* 1547-1553.

Attree, M. (1993). An analysis of the concept "quality" as it relates to contemporary nursing care. *International Journal of Nursing Studies, 30,* 355-369.

Boyd, C. (1985). Toward an understanding of mother-daughter identification using concept analysis. *Advances in Nursing Science,* 78-85.

Campbell, L. (1987). Hopelessness. *Journal of Psychosocial Nursing, 25*(2), 18-29.

Caroline, H. (1993). Explorations of close friendship: A concept analysis. *Archives of Psychiatric Nursing, 7*(4), 236-243.

Chinn, P.L., & Jacobs, M.K. (1983). *Theory and nursing: A systematic approach.* St. Louis, MO: Mosby.

Chinn, P.L., & Jacobs, M.K. (1987). *Theory and nursing: A systematic approach* (2nd ed.). St. Louis, MO: Mosby.

Chinn, P.L., & Kramer, M.K. (1991). *Theory and nursing: A systematic approach.* St. Louis, MO: Mosby Year Book.

Cowles, K. V., & Rodgers, B. L. (1991). The concept of grief: A foundation for nursing research and practice. *Research in Nursing & Health, 14,* 119-127.

Geissler, E. (1984). Crisis: What it is and is not. *Advances in Nursing Science, 6*(4), 1-9.

Gibson, C. (1991). A concept analysis of empowerment. *Journal of Advanced Nursing, 16,* 354-361.

Hagerty, B., Lynch-Sauer, J., Patusky, K., Bouwsema, M., & Collier, P. (1992). Sense of belonging: A vital mental health concept. *Archives of Psychiatric Nursing, 6*(3), 172-177.

Haase, J., Britt, T., Coward, D., Leidy, N. K., & Penn, P. (1992). Simultaneous concept analysis of spiritual perspective, hope, acceptance and self-transcendence. *Image: Journal of Nursing Scholarship, 24*(2), 141-147.

Hawks, J. H. (1991). Power: A concept analysis. *Journal of Advanced Nursing, 16,* 754-762.

Hawks, J. H. (1992). Empowerment in nursing education: Concept analysis and application to philosophy, learning and instruction. *Journal of Advanced Nursing, 17,* 609-618.

Jasper, M. (1994). Expert: A discussion of the implications of the concept as used in nursing. *Journal of Advanced Nursing, 20,* 769-776.

Levine, M. E. (1995). The rhetoric of nursing theory. *Image: Journal of Nursing Scholarship, 27*(1), 11-14.

Lindgren, C., Burke, M., Hainsworth, M., & Eakes, G. (1992). Chronic sorrow: A lifespan concept. *Scholarly Inquiry for Nursing Practice, 6*(1), 27-40.

Madden, B. P. (1990). The hybrid model for concept development: Its value for the study of therapeutic alliance. *Advances in Nursing Science, 12*(3), 75-87.

Mairis, E. (1994). Concept clarification in professional practice—dignity. *Journal of Advanced Nursing, 19,* 947-953.

Matteson, P., & Hawkins, J. (1990). Concept analysis of decision making. *Nursing Forum, 25*(2), 4-10.

Meeberg, G. (1993). Quality of life: A concept analysis. *Journal of Advanced Nursing, 18,* 32-38.

Meize-Grochowski, R. (1984). An analysis of the concept of trust. *Journal of Advanced Nursing, 9,* 563-572.

Nemcek, M. A. (1987). Self nurturing: A concept analysis. *AAOHN Journal, 35*(8), 349-352.

Norris, C. (1982). *Concept clarification in nursing.* Rockville, MD: Aspen .

Phillips, M. (1991). Chronic sorrow in mothers of chronically ill and disabled children. *Issues in Comprehensive Pediatric Nursing, 14,* 111-120.

Reed, P., & Leonard, V. (1989). An analysis of the concept of self-neglect. *Advances in Nursing Science, 12*(1), 39-53.

Rew, L. (1986). Intuition: Concept analysis of a group phenomenon. *Advances in Nursing Science, 8*(2), 21-28.

Reynolds, P. D. (1971). *A primer in theory construction.* Indianapolis, IN: Bobbs-Merill.

Roberts, K., & Fitzgerald, L. (1991). Serenity: Caring with perspective. *Scholarly Inquiry for Nursing Practice, 5*(2), 127-146.

Rodgers, B. L. (1989a). Concepts, analysis and the development of nursing knowledge: The evolutionary cycle. *Journal of Advanced Nursing, 14,* 330-335.

Rodgers, B. L. (1989b). Exploring health policy as a concept. *Western Journal of Nursing Research, 11,* 694-702.

Rodgers, B. L. (1993). Concept analysis: An evolutionary view. In B. L. Rodgers & K. A. Knafl (Eds.), *Concept development in nursing* (pp. 73-106). Philadelphia: Saunders.

Rodgers, B. L., & Cowles, K. V. (1991). The concept of grief: An analysis of classical and contemporary thought. *Death Studies, 15,* 443-458.

Schwartz-Barcott, D., & Kim, H. S. (1986). A hybrid model for concept development. In P.L. Chinn (Ed.), *Nursing research methodology: Issues and implementations* (pp. 91- 101). Rockville, MD: Aspen.

Schwartz-Barcott, D., & Kim, H. S. (1993). An expansion and elaboration of the hybrid model of concept development. In B. L. Rodgers & K. A. Knafl (Eds.), *Concept development in nursing* (pp. 107-133). Philadelphia: Saunders.

Simmons, S. (1989). Health: A concept analysis. *International Journal of Nursing Studies, 26*(2), 155-161.

Schatzman, L., & Strauss, A. L. (1973). *Field research: Strategies for a natural sociology.* Englewood Cliffs, NJ: Prentice Hall.

Stephenson, C. (1991). The concept of hope revisited for nursing. *Journal of Advanced Nursing, 16,* 1456-1461.

Stevens, B. (1984). *Nursing theory: Analysis, application, evaluation* (2nd ed.). Boston: Little, Brown.

Teasdale, K. (1989). The concept of reassurance in nursing. *Journal of Advanced Nursing, 14,* 444-450.

Timmerman, G. (1991). A concept analysis of intimacy. *Issues in Mental Health Nursing, 12,* 19-30.

Verhulst, G., & Schwartz-Barcott, D. (1993) . A concept analysis of withdrawal: Application of the hybrid model of concept development. In B. L. Rodgers & K. A. Knafl (Eds.), *Concept development in nursing* (pp. 135-157). Philadelphia: Saunders.

Walker, L. O., & Avant, K. C. (1983). *Strategies for theory construction in nursing.* Norwalk, CT: Appleton-Century-Crofts.

Walker, L. O., & Avant, K. C. (1988). *Strategies for theory construction in nursing* (2nd ed.). Norwalk, CT: Appleton-Century-Crofts.

Walker, L. O., & Avant, K. C. (1995). *Strategies for theory construction in nursing* (3rd ed.). Norwalk, CT: Appleton-Century-Crofts.

Warren, B. J. (1993). Explaining social isolation through concept analysis. *Archives of Psychiatric Nursing, 7*(5), 270-276.

Watson, S. (1991). An analysis of the concept of experience. *Journal of Advanced Nursing, 16,* 1117-1121.

Westra, B. L., & Rodgers, B. L. (1991). The concept of integration: A foundation for evaluating outcomes of nursing care. *Journal of Professional Nursing, 17,* 277-282.

Wilson, J. (1969). *Thinking with concepts.* Cambridge, England: Cambridge University Press. (Original work published 1963)

2

The Pediatric Physiologic Stress Response: A Concept Analysis

Cathy H. Rosenthal-Dichter, RN, MN, CCRN, FCCM

Pediatric nurses have had a long-standing interest in stress and its effect on infants and children. For over 25 years, research has been conducted on various aspects of the emotional responses of children to the stress of hospitalization and health care (Thompson, 1986). In recent decades, nursing research has expanded to include both the behavioral and the biologic responses to stress and illness (Fagin, 1987) in patients across the life span. This impetus to include a biologic or physiologic component in nursing research is expected to continue since the National Institute of Nursing Research has implemented a 10-year program to increase the use of biologic theory and measurements in nursing through a variety of funding mechanisms (Cowan, Heinrich, Lucas, Sigmon, & Hinshaw, 1993). The incorporation of biologic or physiologic components in nursing research is well suited to critical care settings, such as the pediatric or neonatal intensive care unit, given the nature and complexity of the environment and the availability of information derived from the use of invasive monitoring devices.

In the pediatric critical care setting, nurses continually assess the physiologic stability of the critically ill child as well as the child's responses to a variety of interpersonal interactions, clinical interventions, and treatments. Clinical parameters including, but not limited to, heart rate, respiratory rate, and blood pressure, are often used as barometers of physiologic status. This status is continually challenged by a multitude of stressors which induce subsequent responses by the child. Only through a better understanding of the age-appropriate physiologic stress response can nurses accurately confirm its

Acknowledgment. The author would like to thank Dr. Zoriana Malseed and Dr. Jacqueline Fawcett for their critical review of the manuscript and their support during the Qualifying Examination process.

presence and evaluate its potential consequences. In addition, many nursing interventions are evaluated for tolerance or effectiveness using the patient's physiologic stress response as a criterion. Without an understanding of the physiologic stress response of the neonate, infant, and child, one cannot adequately assess this response in the context of age and clinical condition.

PURPOSE OF THE CONCEPT ANALYSIS

The manifestations of stress include psychologic, behavioral, sociocultural, and physiologic responses (Lindsey, Carrieri-Kohlman, & Page, 1993). For the purpose of this analysis, only the pediatric physiological stress response, hereafter referred to as the stress response, is explored and any reference to the adult stress response is stated explicitly. This concept is selected due to its seemingly complex, ambiguous, and diverse nature noted in the literature and common references to the concept in the clinical arena. The analysis is conducted to clarify the meaning of the concept and its role in the author's program of research. It is intended that the stress response, its attributes, and measurement are illuminated during the analysis.

The process of selecting the method of concept analysis for this study included the following considerations: (1) the author's intent to use a method recommended by nurses and applied to concepts inherent to nursing; (2) the objective, versus subjective, nature of the physiologic concept which impedes the use of a method based on or incorporating qualitative approaches; and (3) congruence between the purposes of this study and the method of analysis to be selected.

This concept analysis begins with an orientation to the concept of stress and stress terminology presented without regard to age or development. After reviewing several methods, the strategy for concept analysis recommended by Walker and Avant (1988) was selected. Accordingly, this analysis will include: (1) a literature review; (2) determination of possible uses of the concept; (3) selection of defining attributes; (4) identification of empirical referents; (5) identification of antecedents and consequences; (6) construction of model and alternative cases; and (7) review of implications for nursing research.

LITERATURE REVIEW

An Orientation to Stress and Stress Terminology

Stress is a prevalent topic in today's society. Stress also is the subject of voluminous research and an ever increasing number of professional publications, conferences, and academic courses. Yet, despite numerous references to the word stress, there is little consensus regarding the meaning or definition of the term (Levine & Ursin, 1991). A commonly cited definition proposed by Selye (1993), generally regarded as the father of the concept (Harris, 1984), is that stress is "the nonspecific result of any demand upon the body" (p. 7). Selye's perspective of stress dictates a response-based definition, with the specific nature of the demand on the body being largely irrelevant (Weiner, 1992).

The multidimensional nature of stress has both facilitated and confounded the process of clarifying the concept of stress. Attempts to clarify a particular dimension of the term stress often result in the elucidation of that dimension's contribution to the concept of stress. The term stressor, in contrast to the word stress, is widely accepted and used to refer to the demand, challenge, or stimulus that elicits a stress response. A mediator or 'filter' is the process whereby an organism evaluates the stressor. Mediators have been the central theme in most contemporary writings on stress (Levine & Ursin, 1991). The stress response is the organism's reaction to the stressor. In sharp contrast to the other dimensions of stress, little is written on the definition of the end product, consequence, or outcome of stress. The challenge surrounding the concept of stress remains, since the dimensions interact with one another (Ursin & Olff, 1993) and the sum of the dimensions fails to adequately represent or clarify the concept of stress.

Illustrations of the dimensions of stress are offered by Levine and Ursin (1991) and by a model presented by the Institute of Medicine (IOM) on Research on Stress and Human Health (Elliot & Eisdorfer, 1982; IOM, 1981). Levine and Ursin (1991) describe stress as comprised of three dimensions: the input (stress stimuli); the processing systems, including the subjective experience of stress; and the output (stress response). The IOM model, as shown in Figure 2.1, depicts stress as comprised of a potential activator (stressor); mediators; and the reaction (the stress response). The IOM model differs from that proposed by Levine and Ursin (1991), as it also illustrates the consequences of the stress response. Whereas the former (Levine & Ursin, 1991) depicts the stress response as the end product of stress, the latter (IOM, 1981) depicts the consequences of stress as an end product, yielding a better representation of the continuum of stress. Consequences are defined as sequelae to the reactions, but of primary interest are changes in health (IOM, 1981). The IOM model diagrammatically represents the stress process as dynamic and sometimes circular, similar to the interactive process that occurs between the organism and the environment (Lowery, 1987). Although the descriptions of the dimensions of stress vary slightly in the literature, there is a congruent trend in the identification of most of the dimensions of stress, as well as in the temporal nature of these dimensions (see Table 2.1).

Selye and the General Adaptation Syndrome

Hans Selye began his pioneering studies of stress in the 1930s. Although during that time the primary impetus in medical science was identification of unique symptomatology, Selye noted the common elements in or reactions to various medical conditions. In a recent retrospective review, Selye (1993) stated "I was struck by how patients suffering from the most diverse diseases exhibited strikingly similar signs and symptoms..." (p. 9). He conceptualized stress as a nonspecific, uniform physiological pattern, consisting of hypertrophy of the adrenal cortex, atrophy of the thymus, spleen, lymph nodes and all other lymphatic structures, and gastric ulceration, occurring as a result of a variety of demands or challenges to an organism (Selye, 1946). These interdependent morphological changes were soon accepted as objective indices of stress. Subsequently, Selye described this nonspecific systemic reaction as one

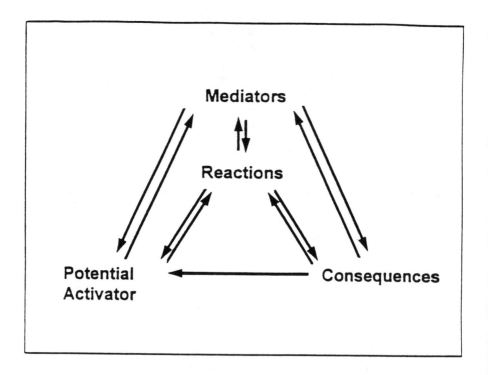

FIGURE 2.1 Model illustrating the dimensions of stress & stress terminology.

(Reprinted with permission from *Research on Stress and Human Health.* Copyright 1981 by the National Academy of Sciences. Courtesy of the National Academy Press, Washington, DC.)

with three stages—alarm, resistance, and exhaustion—which he formally referred to as the General Adaptation Syndrome (GAS) (Selye, 1946, 1993).

The alarm reaction, the initial stage in the GAS, immediately calls into action the body's defensive forces to combat the imposed stressor to which the organism is not adapted. This stage is primarily the function of the sympathetic nervous system (SNS) activation. Cannon (1939) emphasized stimulation of the SNS during his investigations of homeostatic mechanisms and noted that activation of the SNS induces a bodily response which he termed a "fight or flight" response. As shown in Table 2.2, the effects of SNS activation are diverse. The effectors of the "fight or flight " response may be categorized as serving one of two primary functions: maintenance of cardiovascular and pulmonary function and energy or substrate mobilization (Lindsey et al., 1993). Epinephrine is also released from the adrenal medulla in response to SNS activation and serves to prolong and reinforce the "fight or flight" response.

The stage of resistance represents the body's attempts to reestablish stability or adaptation while still in the presence of the stressor. This stage of the stress response reflects the activation of the hypothalamic-pituitary-adrenal (HPA) axis and recruitment of numerous hormones including adrenocorticotrophic hormone (ACTH), glucocorticoids, mineralocorticoids, growth hormone, and antidiuretic hormone (see Table 2.2). The primary end product of the HPA axis is adrenal glucocorticoid release. The catabolic nature of glucocorticoids assists the organism by suppressing immunological responses while increasing the availability of energy substrates, including amino acids and glucose (Rhoades & Pflanzer, 1992). As detailed in Table 2.2, numerous hormones participate in the mobilization and distribution of energy and substrates during this stage of the stress response.

The last stage of the GAS, exhaustion, may occur when a stressor is extremely severe or persists for a sufficient amount of time to consume or deplete the body's reserves and defenses. The stage of exhaustion illustrates the finite nature of the body's ability to respond to a stressor. Selye (1993) stated "[b]ut just as any inanimate machine gradually wears out, so does the

TABLE 2.1 Comparison of the Dimensions of Stress

Levine and Ursin (1991)	IOM Model (IOM, 1981)	Correlates to the Concept Analysis
Input: the stimuli processing variables: input filters	Potential activator Mediators	Antecedent
Outcome variable: stress responses	The reaction	Concept of interest: the stress response
	Consequences	Consequences

TABLE 2.2 Selected Empirical Referents for the Physiologic Stress Response

Sympathetic Nervous System Activation "Fight or Flight Response"	Prepare for Continuation of Stress Response	Hypothalamus-Pituitary- Adrenal Axis Hormone Response
Maintain Cardiovascular Status: Increase HR Increase myocardial force of contraction Increase BP Dilation of coronary & skeletal muscle blood vessels Constriction of cutaneous & visceral vasculature	Increase secretion of catecholamines from adrenal medulla*	Maintain Cardiovascular Status: Increase HR via EPI Increase myocardial force of contraction via EPI Increase BP via EPI Dilation of skeletal muscle blood vessels via EPI Constriction of cutaneous & visceral vasculature via EPI Enhanced vascular responsiveness to catecholamines via GC
Maintain Respiratory Status Relaxation of smooth muscle Increase rate & depth of respiration Provide Sources of Energy: Glycogenolysis in liver & muscle Lipolysis		Maintain Respiratory Status: Relaxation of smooth muscle via EPI Provide Sources of Energy: Glycogenolysis in liver & muscle via EPI Gluconeogenesis via GH, GC Decrease tissue responsiveness to insulin via GH, GC Decrease glucose uptake in adipose & muscle via GH, GC Increase glycogen synthesis via EPI, GH Lipolysis via EPI, GH, GC Oxidation of fatty acids via GC Protein degradation via GC
Maintain Blood Volume: Enhance blood coagulation Contraction of spleen Enhance CNS Alertness		Maintain Blood Volume: Increase Na retention via aldosterone Increase H2O reabsorption via ADH Enhance CNS Alertness: Stimulate mental alertness via EPI

Key: NS—Sympthetic Nervous System; HR—heart rate; BP—blood pressure; GI—gastrointestinal; EPI—epinephrine; Na—sodium; H_2O—water; GH—growth hormone; GC—gluocorticoids (e.g., cortisol). *Release of catecholamines from the adrenal medulla is a result of SNS activation, but is positioned in the table between the two columns to represent the role of catecholamines in reinforcing and prolonging the fight or flight response.

human machine sooner or later become the victim of constant wear and tear" (p. 10). Metaphorically, Selye (1993) equated the three stages of the GAS with three stages of the human life cycle: *childhood*, characterized by low resistance and an excessive response to any kind of stimulus (alarm stage); *adulthood*, characterized by an increased resistance and adaptation to the most commonly encountered agents; and *senility*, characterized by the loss of adaptation and eventual exhaustion (and death).

Possible Uses of the Concept

Although references to the adult physiologic stress response abound in the literature, references to pediatric physiologic stress response are more limited (Doswell, 1989). Most references to the concept of interest involve scant descriptions of the concept or a reiteration of what is known of the adult response with a brief discussion of the proposed differences that may exist between patients at different stages of development (Stidham & Bugnitz, 1992). A seminal review of the neonate's response to operative stress, conducted by Schmeling and Coran (1991), proved the most comprehensive. Although this review is comprehensive in one instance, it was limited in scope with regard to the type of stressor (surgical) and age (neonate).

Given the various disciplines concerned with the concept of interest, this author felt it was imperative to examine interdisciplinary applicable literature. This step in the analysis represents a departure from recommendations made by Walker and Avant (1988). There are differences among different disciplines, such as nursing, psychology, and medicine, with regard to conceptual framework, terminology of and references to the concept, intent of the research, and the type and frequency of empirical referents. These differences, which reflect the discipline's philosophy or worldview of stress and of the pediatric physiological stress response, are summarized in Table 2.3.

ATTRIBUTES, EMPIRICAL REFERENTS, ANTECEDENTS, AND CONSEQUENCES

Attributes

Attributes are defining characteristics or salient features that assist in identifying the occurrence of the concept. Attributes of the stress response emerged as consistent themes upon review of the literature and in the examination of the model cases. The stress response is not an undesirable or atavistic response, but one that is an integral part of an adaptive biological system. It is considered protective, in fact, the stress response is categorized as a protective life process by Carrieri-Kohlman and colleagues (1993) in their textbook entitled *Pathophysiological Phenomena in Nursing*. It is categorized as such since the stress

TABLE 2.3 Comparison of the Concept of the Pediatric Physiologic Stress Response in Nursing, Psychology, and Medical Literature

Concept Characteristic	Nursing Literature	Psychology Literature	Medical Literature
Terminology Used for Concept	Physiologic arousal, Physiologic response, Psychophysiologic effects.	Adrenocorticoid response, cortisol response, physiologic responsivity, physiologic indicators of distress	Endocrine response, hormonal response, cortisol response, sympathoadrenal response, metabolic response
Conceptual Framework	Infrequent references to: Selye Cannon	Some references to: Selye	Some references to: Selye
Philosophy/World View	Organismic[1]	Organismic[1]	Mechanistic[1]
Purpose of Research	To describe a patient's actual or potential response to phenomena including: pain hospitalization parental presence/anxiety preprocedural/preoperative preparation	To describe the infant or child's response to: maternal separation hospitalization, preprocedural/ preoperative preparation	To describe the mechanism of the pediatric physiological stress response or components thereof. To contrast the response of the neonate and pediatric patient to the response of the adult patient. To explore methods of mitigating the response.
Type & Frequency of Empiric Referent	Varies from study to study. Predominantly noninvasive end organ effects or indicators such as heart rate, blood pressure, etc. Usually collected several times (3–5) in a repeated measures design.	Varies from study to study. Both hormone as well as end organ effects or indicators of response. Cortisol (serum and salivary) was common. Usually collected several times (2–3) in a repeated measures design.	Varies from study to study. A wide variety of specific hormones and metabolic substrates are collected. Usually collected many times (5–7) during the research protocol that may extend up to 72 hours.

[1]The organicism-mechanism dichotomy illustrates the divergent characteristics of two world views or philosophies to the study of the human-environment relationship. A few characteristics of organistic worldview include holism and expansionism and development that is quantitative and qualitative, whereas mechanistic worldview include elementarism and reductionism and development that is quantitative (Fawcett, 1993).

response assists in shielding the organism from stressors and altering the impact of stressors (Carrieri-Kohlman et al., 1993). The response, including the behavioral and physiological components, is necessary to the functioning and survival of the organism in a dynamic, complex environment (Ursin & Olff, 1993).

Activation of the stress response occurs when there is an imbalance in or challenge to the environment of the organism (Lindsey et al., 1993; Ursin & Olff, 1993). This activation serves as a warning system (or alarm), as well as the driving force that forces the organism to act to redirect energy and function during a time of need. The response is also graded, rather than an all or none response. Ursin and Olff (1993) state:

> ... when there is a discrepancy between the set value and the actual value for a particular variable, the alarm system or driving force will remain activated until there is an agreement between them, or until the brain gives a lower priority to the set value. (p. 9)

The composite of interrelated and interdependent neuroendocrine and metabolic events that comprise the stress response reflects the coordinating and integrating roles of the brain. The brain not only controls the autonomic nervous system, but also the central nervous system influences on stress response effectors, leading to endocrine, metabolic, and immunological responses (Ursin & Olff, 1993). The magnitude and duration of the stress response, even to the same stressor, varies from individual to individual. Mediator processes are primarily responsible for this lack of linearity between the stressor and the stress response. This relationship between the stressor and the stress response is influenced by mediators, since the stressor is processed and evaluated before it gains access to the response (effector) system (Ursin & Olff, 1993). Mediators are generally categorized as those that evaluate the stressor and those that evaluate the resources to deal with the stressor (Ursin & Olff, 1993).

Consistent characteristics of the concept, derived through the review of the literature and the examination of the model cases, were assembled. Additionally, the "characteristics" of the [adult] stress response, as identified by Lindsey and colleagues (1993), assisted this author in refining attributes for this concept analysis. Attributes of the stress response, whether pediatric or adult, include the following:

The stress response begins as a normal, protective, and adaptive response to stressors.

The stress response is a graded, not an all or none, response.

The stress response consists of a composite of interrelated and interdependent neuroendocrine and metabolic events.

The magnitude and duration of the stress response, even to the same stressor, varies from individual to individual.

The magnitude and duration of the stress response can be influenced by multidisciplinary interventions.

Empirical Referents

Empirical referents demonstrate how the concept exists in the real world and how the concept is measured (Rew, 1986; Walker & Avant, 1988). Empirical referents demonstrate the unquestionable existence of the concept through observable, measurable, and verifiable means. The classic signs and symptoms of the "fight or flight" response are empiric referents of the physiologic stress response since these may be observed, measured, and verified. Other examples of empirical referents abound in the literature and include all hormones and their precursors, metabolic substrates, and other endogenous mediators (i. e., opioids, prostaglandins, cytokines) involved in any aspect of the physiologic stress response. Empirical referents of the concept of interest vary greatly in the level of specificity (receptors versus hormones versus physiologic parameters such as heart rate) as well as origin (e.g., serum, urinary, or salivary). Examples of other empirical referents can be found in Tables 2.2 and 2.3, as well as in the model and borderline cases presented in this analysis.

Antecedents and Consequences

Antecedents are the incidents that occur prior to the concept of interest, whereas consequences are the result of the concept of interest. It is through the identification of the antecedents and consequences that the attributes of the concept become clearer, because attributes can be neither antecedents nor consequences (Walker & Avant, 1988). Antecedents of the stress response include all events, actual or perceived, that stimulate or induce such a response from the child. In other words, antecedents include any and all stressors. Antecedents are diverse in nature (physiologic and psychologic), duration, frequency, and intensity. Although it is beyond the scope of this concept analysis to list all possible stressors, common physiologic stressors for the pediatric critical care patient include sepsis, tissue injury (surgery or trauma), and respiratory infection (Yeh, 1992). Psychological stressors for the pediatric critical care patient include separation from parents, presence of unfamiliar personnel, and the complexity of critical care equipment and environment (Kidder, 1989; Wilson & Broome, 1989). Congruent with the notion that stress is more than a stimulus response, it is important to note that mediators (e.g., processes of cognitive appraisal and coping) may intensify a stress response if the stressor is evaluated as extraordinarily dangerous or if it is evaluated that there is an imbalance between the demand and the resources to attend to the demand.

Consequences include temporary and/or permanent conditions that occur as a result of the concept of interest (Walker & Avant, 1988). Given the lack of definition and clarity regarding the outcome dimension of stress, referred to earlier in this paper, it is no surprise that the identification of consequences to the stress response would be challenging. The stress response is considered an integral part of an adaptive biological system; consequently it is inherently considered a benign event with a salient purpose. Therefore, the consequence, in some instances, is optimal and results in the resolution of the stressor, the cessation of the stress response, and restoration of physiologic stability. There are also references in the literature to pathological consequences of the stress response. These consequences of the stress response have been noted for clinical states, such as the common cold, asthmatic attacks, anorexia nervosa, and obesity (Chrousos & Gold, 1992; Dorn & Chrousos, 1993; Lindsey et al., 1993). Pathophysiologic consequences appear to be associated with prolonged activation of the stress response (Ursin & Olff, 1993). The relationship between the stress response and these clinical states, however, is one of association rather than causation (Lindsey et al., 1993).

Consequences of the stress response may be more detrimental in neonatal and pediatric patients due to their relative immaturity and their documented anatomical and physiological differences from older patients. Neonatal and pediatric patients are prone to metabolic instability due to (1) a greater body surface area necessitating greater heat production; (2) a larger brain-to-body-weight ratio, with increased obligatory glucose requirements; (3) a need to maintain somatic growth; and (4) relatively smaller reserves of protein, carbohydrate, and fat (Anand & Ward-Platt, 1988). These developmental differences are greater in the neonate and decrease gradually with increasing age, yet they continue to exist to some degree throughout childhood.

MODEL AND ALTERNATIVE CASES

Model Cases

Model cases best represent the concept of interest and assist in the identification of the essential features of a concept (Avant, 1993). Although model cases may be fabricated patient situations or accumulations of information depicting ideal case studies (Goosen, 1989), the author strived to inductively select model cases relevant to the context of nursing and derived from the scientific literature. It is perceived that model cases with these characteristics would best fulfill the purpose in conducting this concept analysis. This step represents a modification of the process recommended by Walker and Avant (1988) in that cases are usually deductively constructed to illustrate the concept's attributes.

Examination of nursing studies or programs of research failed to identify a model case that exhibited the attributes of the concept of interest. Model cases presented in this concept analysis are extrapolated from research reports from medical programs of research conducted by Anand and colleagues (Anand & Hickey, 1992; Anand, Sippell, & Aynsley-Green, 1987) and other researchers exploring the stress responses of children to operative stressors (Wolf et al.,

1993). Although the model cases were extrapolated from research addressing medical questions, the same methodology can be applied to answer nursing questions. For example, relevant studies would be the examination of the stress responses of children receiving two different nursing interventions or the effects of parental presence and separation on the stress responses of children in the pediatric intensive care unit.

Each of the model cases investigated the stress responses of children to operative stressors and is summarized in greater detail in Table 2.4. Three model cases are presented to illustrate the pediatric physiologic stress response across the continuum of development. These studies were randomized clinical trials that involved controlled, uniform surgical techniques and protocol-directed preoperative, perioperative, and postoperative care. A variety of serum hormones and metabolites, urinary metabolites, and indices of clinical course were collected throughout the protocols. Researchers then compared preoperative, perioperative and postoperative values of the selected empiric referents.

Model Case # 1. Anand and colleagues (1987) compared the operative stress responses of preterm neonates receiving different anesthetic regimens. Responses of the control group receiving a conventional anesthetic regimen were compared to responses of a treatment group, receiving fentanyl in addition to the conventional anesthesia. Comparison of preoperative, perioperative and postoperative values revealed multiple hormonal responses to the operative stressor in both the control and treatment groups. In general, hormonal responses were significantly greater in the control group as compared to the treatment group. Although there were no significant differences between the two groups in cortisol responses, precursors to cortisol (corticosterone and 11-deoxycortisol) were significantly greater in the control group as compared to the treatment group. Significant differences in metabolic responses, specifically glucose, lactate, and pyruvate, were also noted between the groups. Although the differences in clinical course were not subjected to statistical analyses, the control group experienced more postoperative complications compared to the treatment group.

Model Case #2. Anand and Hickey (1992) compared the operative stress responses of full-term term neonates receiving different anesthetic regimens. Responses of the control group, receiving a conventional anesthetic regimen were compared to responses of a treatment group, receiving high-dose suffentanil. Comparison of preoperative, perioperative and postoperative values revealed major hormonal responses to the operative stressor in both the control and treatment groups. In general, hormonal responses, including cortisol responses, were significantly greater in the control group as compared to the treatment group. Significant differences in metabolic responses, specifi-

TABLE 2.4 Studies Comprising the Model Cases for the Pediatric Physiologic Stress Response

Study/Conceptual Framework	Purpose/ Subjects	Methodology/ Stressor	Measures/ Definition	Findings
Wolf, Eyres, Laussen, Edwards, Stanley, Row, & Simon, 1993 Conceptual Framework: None specified	Purpose: To investigate the effects of extradural anesthesia/analgesia versus opioid anasthesia/analgesia on the child's stress response. Sample: $N = 40$, Children: ages 2 months to 4 years	Design: Experimental (randomized clinical trial) Randomized to receive general anasthesia supplemented during and after sugery with either: systemic opioids extradural bupivacaine Stressor Elective, major abdominal surgery	Measues: Measured the following serum hormone levels at baseline, 45 minutes after the start of surgery, 1 hour and 24 hours after the end of surgery: epinephrine (EPI) norepinephrine (NE) glucose adrenocorticotrophic (ACTH) cortisol Bupivacaine levels in patients receiving bupivacaine were also measured at same intervals. Definitions: None specified for the study concepts	Baseline measures were within normal range. Patient characteristics were similar between groups. Perioperative increases in EPI, glucose and ACTH were significantly greater in the opioid group as compared to the extradural group. NE concentration did not change significantly during or after surgery in opioid group, but in extradural group they were significantly less than those in opioid group. The perioperative increase in cortisol was similar between the groups despite the difference noted in ACTH. ACTH increased in both groups during surgery, but was significantly greater in the opioid group.
Anand & Hickey, 1992 Conceptual Framework: None specified	Purpose: To investigate the effects of deep opioid anesthesia on the stress responses and clinical outcome of critically ill neonates.	Design: Experimental (randomized clinical trial) Randomized to receive general anesthesia supplemented during and	Measures: Measured the following serum hormonal and metabolic substrate levels at six sampling points (at the end of the operation and	No significant differences noted preoperatively. Suffentanil group had significantly, reduced responses of beta-endorphin, NE, EPI, glucagon, aldosterone, cortisol, and other steroid hormones.

TABLE 2.4 (Continued)

Study/Conceptual Framework	Purpose/ Subjects	Methodology/ Stressor	Measures/ Definition	Findings
	Subjects: $N = 45$, Neonates, term	after surgery with either: halothane-morphine high dose suffentanil/fentanyl Stressor: Cardiac surgery including cardiopulmonary bypass and hypothermic cardiac arrest. Neonates experienced a variety of corrective or palliative repairs of congenital heart defects, such as transposition of the great vessels and Tetralogy of Fallot.	at 6, 12, and 24 hours following the operation) after the preoperative baseline: EPI and NE, glucose, steroid hormones, insulin, glucagon, beta-endorphin, lactate and pyruvate, acetacetate, 3-hydroxy-butyrate, alanine Outcome data was also recorded and included: postoperative mortality and morbidity, hypotension, atrial or ventricular arrhythmias, sepsis, DIC, and seizures Definitions: Operationally defined outcome criteria	Suffentanil group had greater insulin responses and greater insulin:glucagon ratios during the operation. Halothane-morphine group had more severe hyperglycemia and lactic acidemia during surgery and higher lactate and acetoacetate concentrations postoperatively. Suffentanil group had lower incidence of sepsis, metabolic acidosis, DIC, and postoperative deaths than the halothane-morphine group. 4 of the 15 in the halothane-morphine group died whereas none of the 30 in the suffentanil group died.
Anand, Sippell, & Aynsley-Green, 1987 Conceptual Framework: None specified	Purpose: To compare the surgical stress responses of pre term babies receiving two different anesthesia regimens.	Design: Experimental (randomized clinical trial) Randomized to receive either: anesthesia with nitrous oxide &	Measures: Measured the following serum hormonal and metabolic substrate levels at six sampling points (at the end of the operation and at 6, 12, and 24	No significant differences between the groups preoperatively. Hormonal responses to surgery were significantly greater in the non-fentanyl group than the fentanyl group as indicated by

(Continued)

TABLE 2.4 (Continued)

Study/Conceptual Framework	Purpose/ Subjects	Methodology/ Stressor	Measures/ Definition	Findings
	Subjects: $N = 16$ Neonates, preterm	curare alone anesthesia with nitrous oxide & curare & fentanyl Stressor: Operative repair of the PDA	hours following the operation) after the preoperative baseline: EPI and NE, glucose, steroid hormones, insulin, glucagon, beta-endorphin, lactate and pyruvate, acetate, 3-hydroxybutyrate, alanine, triglycerides and glycerol Concentrations of 3-methylhistadine and creatinine in the urine (3MH/Cr) were also measured. Clinical course was also assessed to include: heart rate, respiratory support, incidence of bradycardia, peripheral circulation, oliguria, GI bleeding, metabolic acidosis, and paralytic ileus. Definitions: None specified for the study concepts	changes in EPI, NE, glucagon, aldosterone, insulin/glucagon ratio, blood glucose, lactate, and pyruvate levels. There were no significant differences in cortisol between the two groups, however, corticosterone and 11-deoxycortisol responses were significantly greater in the no-fentanyl group than in the fentanyl group. Compared to the fentanyl group, the no-fentanyl group had circulatory and metabolic complications noted postoperatively. No-fentanyl group was more likely to require an increase in ventilatory support. Two neonates in the no-fentanyl group developed IVH.

Note. IVH = Intraventricular hemorrahage; PDA = Patent ductus arteriosus

cally glucose and lactate, were also noted between the groups. Statistically significant differences were noted in the clinical course and outcome between the groups, with the treatment group experiencing a lower incidence of complications and mortality.

Model Case # 3. Wolf and colleagues (1993) compared the stress responses of children ages 2 months to 4 years receiving extradural anesthesia to those of children receiving opioid anesthesia/analgesia while undergoing elective abdominal surgery. As reported in preterm (Anand et al., 1987) and term neonates (Anand & Hickey, 1992), the results of this study (Wolf et al., 1993) indicated that there were major hormonal responses in both groups to the operative stressor. All measured hormones, with the exception of norepinephrine (NE), increased significantly in both groups during surgery. In general, hormonal responses were significantly greater in the control group than the treatment group, as indicated by epinephrine, glucose, and ACTH. Although NE concentrations did not change significantly during or after surgery in either group, the treatment group had significantly lower NE levels than children in the control group. No group differences were found for cortisol, despite differences in ACTH responses.

Discussion of Model Cases. All attributes of the pediatric physiologic stress response are illustrated in these model cases, including the ability to mitigate the physiologic stress response with interventions, specifically anesthetic regimens. The stress responses were induced as normal, adaptive, and protective responses to the operative stressor. Although summary measures are presented in the research reports, standard errors of the mean reflect the variance of individual responses in that measure and the graded response of each subject. The monitoring of the wide variety of hormones and metabolites used in these model cases facilitates the identification of a composite of hormonal and metabolic events.

These model cases illustrate not only that the response magnitude and duration vary from individual to individual, but also that they vary with the age or development of the patient, making these attributes applicable to individuals across the life span. Although it is beyond the scope of this concept analysis to comprehensively describe the quantitative and qualitative differences noted in the stress response across the continuum of development, a few differences are illustrated in the research that comprises the model cases. In general, hormonal responses of both the neonatal and older pediatric patients are greater in magnitude and shorter in duration than the responses of adults to similar procedures (Anand & Ward-Platt, 1988). Differences are also noted in the response of the preterm and term neonate. The most notable of these differences illustrated in the model cases is the cortisol response. In order to best evaluate the preterm infant's plasma steroid hormone response, steroid precursor hormones, including progesterone, 17-hydroxyprogesterone, 11-deoxycorticosterone, and 11-deoxycortisol, need to be taken into consideration. Term neonates respond with significantly greater cortisol during and after surgery, whereas preterm neonates respond with significantly greater precursor steroid hormones (Anand & Ward-Platt, 1988). Preterm neonates exhibit a relative immaturity for steroid biosynthesis (Solomon, Bird, Ling, Iwamiya, & Young, 1967). Inasmuch as maturation of the hydroxylase enzymes occurs from the proximal to distal end of the steroid biosynthetic pathway (Solomon et al., 1967), the preterm neonate will display a diminished secretion of the final products of steroid biosynthesis (e.g., cortisol) and increased secretion of the precursor steroid hormones (Anand et al., 1987).

Borderline Cases

Borderline cases are those cases that cause difficulty in determining whether they are examples of the concept of interest. By understanding why these cases are difficult to classify, one can further clarify the concept of interest (Avant, 1993). The borderline cases presented in this concept analysis are extrapolated from nursing research and from a series of studies within a program of psychology research conducted by Gunnar and colleagues (Gunnar, Connors, Isensee, & Wall, 1988; Gunnar, Hertsgaard, Larson, & Rigatuso, 1992a). The two borderline cases are classified as such for different reasons.

Borderline Case # 1. Acute pain is an example of a borderline case for the pediatric physiologic stress response. Nurse researchers have investigated several physiologic indicators of acute pain. According to Hester (1993), these studies were based upon the following axioms: (1) Stress arousal alters physiologic responses; (2) pain is a stress arousal; and (3) physiologic responses change with the presence of pain. The pediatric physiologic parameters examined in relationship to acute pain include changes in body temperature (Abu-Saad, 1984; Abu-Saad & Holzemer, 1981); heart rate or pulse (Abu-Saad, 1984; Abu-Saad & Holzemer, 1981; Dale, 1986; Froese-Fretz, 1986; Johnston & Strada, 1986; Mills, 1989); respiratory rate (Abu-Saad, 1984; Abu-Saad & Holzemer, 1981; Mills, 1989); blood pressure (Abu-Saad, 1984; Abu-Saad & Holzemer, 1981); transcutaneous oxygen ($TcpO_2$) (Froese-Fretz, 1986; Norris, Campbell, & Brenkert, 1982); skin color (Mills, 1989); and diaphoresis (Mills, 1989). These studies have yielded inconsistent results. The findings differ according to the type of pain (pain associated with tissue injury or surgery versus pain associated with medical procedures) and show a great degree of variability among individuals in the physiologic response to pain (Hester, 1993). Hester (1993) proposed that the changes in physiologic parameters may have occurred with other stress-arousing events (confounding variables) limiting these parameters as measures of pain. In addition, the relationship between physiologic responses, such as those measured by nurse researchers investigating pain, and neurohormonal and metabolic events has yet to be fully defined. Craig and Grunau (1993) point out that ". . . physiologic events are multidetermined. They can vary with a multitude of physiological and psychological events" (p. 82).

One could argue that acute pain illustrates most of the defining attributes of the stress response. The definition of pain, according to the International Association for the Study of Pain (Merskey et al., 1979) is

> . . . an unpleasant sensory and emotional experience associated with actual or potential tissue damage, or described in terms of such damage. [Note: Pain is always subjective. Each individual learns the application of the word through experiences related to injury early in life. . .](p. 250).

This definition reflects the multidimensional nature of the concept of acute pain. Acute pain may share most of the defining attributes of the stress response, but it most probably has additional defining attributes that would distinguish it from the stress response. Nursing research has reflected the notion that pain is an antecedent to the stress response. It may be more accurate in many cases to state that tissue damage, rather than pain, is an antecedent to the stress response. Further examination of the defining attributes of acute pain would be required before classifying it as a contrary or model case. Thus, acute pain is classified as a borderline case.

Borderline Case #2. Gunnar and colleagues have conducted several studies to examine the adrenocortical and behavioral responses of neonates and infants to various stressors including: limb restraints (Malone, Gunnar, & Fisch, 1985), circumcision, blood sampling, weighing, and physical examination (Gunnar et al., 1988), and repeated stressors (Gunnar et al., 1992a). Studies conducted early in this program of research involved the collection procedures and validation that the two sources of cortisol showed acceptable correlation, investigators used only salivary cortisol in subsequent research.

There have been increases in both serum and salivary cortisol that document the infant's response to stressors, specifically to noxious nociceptive and handling stressors. In response to noxious nociceptive stressors (heelsticks and circumcision), the elevation in serum cortisol was also associated with how much a baby cries, but no such association was found with the stress of handling (Gunnar et al., 1988). These cortisol responses showed sensitization to heelsticks and habituation to discharge examinations in healthy newborns (Gunnar et al., 1988, 1992a). However, a different pattern of response was noted in newborns who were considered in "nonoptimal health." Although these newborns showed sensitization to the repeated heelsticks, they failed to show habituation to the discharge exam (Gunnar et al., 1992a). Furthermore, in "nonoptimal health" newborns, crying was associated with an increase in salivary cortisol with both nociceptive stressors and handling stressors (Gunnar, 1992, 1992a).

Studies involving older infants have included examination of salivary cortisol responses to distress-producing events, including separation from mother (Gunnar, Larson, Hertsgaard, Harris, Brodersen, 1992b; Gunnar, Mangelsdorf, Larson, Hertsgaard, 1989; Larson, Gunnar, & Hertsgaard, 1991). Larson and colleagues (1991) found significant increases in cortisol during separation as compared to a 30-minute play session with the mother. These infants, when separated, were left with a baby-sitter who responded to the infants when they cried, but otherwise interacted minimally with the infants. Interestingly, a recent study (Gunnar et al., 1992b) with a baby-sitter who was responsive to the infants when they cried, but also interacted and played with the infants, completely buffered this cortisol response to separation. Gunnar and colleagues (1992b) have proposed that the quality of care received during the mother-infant separation influences the intensity of the stress response.

Although most attributes are present in this borderline case, the measure of a single hormonal response may not be sufficient to document the stress response. The cortisol alone does not represent a composite of interrelated and interdependent neuroendocrine and metabolic responses. Since only one hormone was measured, this program of research best illustrates a borderline case.

IMPLICATIONS TO NURSING RESEARCH

In summary, what is currently known about the pediatric physiologic stress response is derived from numerous studies from various disciplines using different conceptual frameworks and methodologies. It is essential to combine disciplinary resources to capture a broad and comprehensive view of the concept of interest and its short-term and long-term consequences. The continuum of the stress response to medical and operative stressors also requires further investigation. Several studies investigating the concept in response to operative stress captured the initiation and beginning dissipation of the alarm stage of the GAS. Nonetheless, several key questions remain unanswered. Does the stress response continue to dissipate postoperatively? Are there events or nursing interventions that mitigate the stress response postoperatively? How does the stress response to operative stressors compare to that seen with medical stressors? The stress response associated with medical stressors is proposed to differ from operative stressors, given the discrete time frame and degree of control associated with the latter. Which nursing interventions mitigate or exacerbate the stress response associated with medical stressors?

There are several implications of this concept analysis for nursing research. It is imperative that a conceptual framework be included in future research regarding the pediatric physiologic stress response and that there be consistency between the framework and the research hypothesis and methodology. Clarification as to whether the physiologic stress response or an antecedent, empiric referent, or consequence of the physiologic stress response will be the concept of interest in a study is essential.

Implications for nursing research in regard to empirical referents of the physiologic stress response exist as well. How many hormones or metabolic substrates should be measured to consider the data reflective of a composite neuroendocrine and metabolic event? Measuring only one of the hormones or metabolic substrates in isolation is not sufficient to represent the concept and may leave some degree of doubt as to the body's response. Since the stress response is a graded, not an all or none event, it can exist with wide variation in intensity. A baseline assessment of the patient may more accurately determine the existence and degree of intensity of the stress response. The collection of accurate baseline data can verify the existence of the stress response, as well as assist in the identification of factors that may mask (e.g., beta adrenergic blocking agents) or imitate (e.g., exogenous catecholamine administration) the stress response. In addition to using baseline observations, comparisons of the empirical referent to an accepted and a priori standard assist in the accurate interpretation of the value obtained. Although Guzzetta and Forsyth (1979) were interested in determining parameters that were sensitive and clinically useful in the concept of stress rather than the stress response, they developed a priori operational definitions for selected physiological parameters. For instance, the characteristic of the physiological parameter, heart rate, that defined the existence of stress was a rise of greater than 10 beats per minute over three observation periods (Guzzetta & Forsyth, 1979). There is difficulty in determining the level at which the stress response is considered present. The existence and degree of intensity along a continuum is challenging without the use of baseline observations or comparison to an accepted or a priori standard. Of equal importance, the physiologic stress response must be considered in light of statistical as well as clinical significance. It behooves the researcher, as well as the clinician, to determine the criteria for determining presence, clinical, and statistical significance in an a priori fashion.

The implications regarding consequences of the stress response are numerous. There is a need to examine the relationship between the outcome dimension of stress and the consequences of stress response. Little discussion of the consequences of the concept exists in the literature. In addition, minimal distinctions between short- and long-term consequences are found. Whereas sustained activation of the stress response may contribute to some of the clinical states cited in the literature such as the common cold, it most probably does not account for the differences in clinical outcome illustrated by the model cases presented in this analysis.

There appear to be two dichotomous views in the literature regarding the nature of the concept and its consequences: (1) the stress response is benign and the outcomes can range from optimal to pathologic; (2) both the stress response and the outcomes can range from optimal to pathologic. The IOM (1981) report states "[s]tressors, reactions, and mediators are neither 'good' or 'bad'; only consequences can appropriately be qualified as being desirable or undesirable" (p. 22). Although the majority of the literature is consistent with this philosophy, a recent proposition suggests otherwise. It is proposed that stress response dysfunction, characterized by sustained hyperactivity or hypoactivity, leads to pathophysiologic consequences including the presence or the susceptibility to a wide range of psychiatric, endocrine, and inflammatory disorders (i. e., posttraumatic stress disorder) (Chrousos & Gold, 1992; Dorn & Chrousos, 1993). Again, these are long-term consequences, but what, if any, are the short-term consequences of stress response dysfunction?

The elements of the difference between the physiologic and pathophysiologic stress response have plagued the inquisitive nature of many researchers and clinicians. Anand (1993) proposed factors that are associated with the actual or potential risk of a pathologic stress response. These include: (1) patient vulnerability; (2) magnitude of the response; (3) duration of the response; and (4) conditions exacerbating the stress response or its detrimental effects.

The examination of related cases would assist in the identification of the network of concepts of which the concept of interest is a part. It is through this examination that one can understand how the concept is the same and how it is different from those in the same network (Avant, 1993). For this analysis, although related cases were not developed, it should be noted that knowledge of related concepts and creation of related cases can be helpful in analyzing the concept of interest. In particular, the concepts of stability (or instability) and adaptation are most probably in the same network as the concept of interest. Although critical care clinicians commonly refer to patients as stable or unstable, references in the literature to the concept of stability primarily relate to an instrument measuring severity of illness, the Physiologic Stability Index (Pollack, Ruttiman, Getson, 1988; Ruttiman, Albert, Pollack, & Glass, 1986; Yeh, 1992). Gorski (1983) and other neonatal clinicians use the concept of stability and its contrary term (instability) in discussions of the preterm neonate's neurobehavioral immaturity and disorganization, although the lack of clarity of the concept remains. With regard to the concept of adaptation, Goosen and Bush (1979) reported a concept analysis and viewed adaptation as a 5-step process following the perception of the stimulus that included: (1) cognitive appraisal; (2) coping mechanism; (3) neurophysiological arousal; (4) emotional and physiologic response; and (5) intensification of neurophysiological and psychological response. At each step in the process the individual has the opportunity to continue in the process or to adapt. The conclusion from the concept analysis of adaptation is that this concept encompasses the concept of physiologic stress response. How the concepts of adaptation and stability differ from the physiologic stress response requires further investigation.

Lastly, examination of the pediatric physiologic stress response within a nursing context is integral to the determination of the degree and direction of the child's responses to interpersonal interaction, clinical interventions, and treatment. Investigations must include a clear conceptual-theoretical-empirical structure that accurately defines the role of the concept of interest within that study. It behooves the nurse researcher to maintain an organismic perspective during such investigations, since it is human responses that are of interest and importance to nurses. Wolf (1993) titled a recent editorial "[T]reat the babies, not their stress responses," as a mere reminder of the importance in placing these investigations within the context of patient outcomes.

REFERENCES

Abu-Saad, H. (1984). Assessing children's responses to pain. *Pain, 19*, 163-171.

Abu-Saad, H., & Holzemer, W. L. (1981). Measuring children's self-assessment of pain. *Issues in Comprehensive Pediatric Nursing, 5,* 337-349.

Anand, K. J. S. (1993). Relationships between stress responses and clinical outcome in newborns, infants, and children. *Critical Care Medicine, 21*(9), S358-S359.

Anand, K. J. S., & Hickey, P. R. (1992). Halothane-morphine compared to high dose sufentanil for anesthesia and postoperative analgesia in neonatal cardiac surgery. *New England Journal of Medicine, 326,* 1-9.

Anand, K. J. S., Sippell, W. G., & Aynsley-Green, A. (1987). Randomized trial of fentanyl anaesthesia in preterm babies undergoing surgery: Effects on the stress response. *The Lancet, 1,* 243-248.

Anand, K. S., & Ward-Platt, M. P. (1988). Neonatal and pediatric stress responses to anesthesia and operation. *International Anesthesiology Clinics, 26*(3), 218-225.

Avant, K. C. (1993). The Wilson method of concept analysis. In B. L. Rodgers & K. A. Knafl (Eds.), *Concept development in nursing: Foundations, techniques, and applications* (pp. 51-72). Philadelphia: W. B. Saunders Company.

Cannon, W. B. (1939). *The wisdom of the body.* Philadelphia: W. W. Norton.

Carrieri-Kohlman, V., Lindsey, A. M., & West, C. M. (1993). Alterations in protection. In V. Carrieri-Kohlman, A. M. Lindsey, & C. M. West (Eds.), *Pathophysiological phenomena in nursing: Human responses to illness* (2nd ed., pp. 395-396). Philadelphia: W. B. Saunders Company.

Chrousos, G. P., & Gold, P. W. (1992). The concepts of stress and stress system disorders: Overview of physical and behavioral homeostasis. *Journal of the American Medical Association, 267*(9), 1244-1252.

Cowan, M. J., Heinrich, J., Lucas, M., Sigmon, H., & Hinshaw, A. S. (1993). Integration of biological and nursing sciences: A 10-year plan to enhance research and training. *Research in Nursing & Health, 16,* 3-9.

Craig, K. D., & Grunau, R. V. E. (1993). Neonatal pain perception and behavioral measurement. In K. J. S. Anand & P. J. McGrath (Eds)., *Pain in neonates* (pp. 67-105). Amsterdam: Elsevier.

Dale, J. C. (1986). A multidimensional study of infants' responses to painful stimuli. *Pediatric Nursing, 12*, 31-37.

Dorn, L. D., & Chrousos, G. P. (1993). The endocrinology of stress and stress system disorders in adolescence. *Endocrinology and Metabolism Clinics of North America, 22*(2), 685-700.

Doswell, W. (1989). Physiological responses to stress. *Annual Review of Nursing Research, 7,* 51-69.

Elliot, G., & Eisdorfer, C. (1982). *Stress and human health.* New York: Springer Publishing Company.

Fagin, C. M. (1987). Stress: Implications for nursing research. *Image: Journal of Nursing Scholarship, 19*(1), 4-38.

Fawcett, J. (1993). The structure of contemporary nursing knowledge. In J. Fawcett, *Analysis and evaluation of nursing theories* (pp. 1-3). Philadelphia: F. A. Davis.

Froese-Fretz, A. (1986). The use of transcutaneous electrical nerve stimulators (TENS) during radial arterial blood sampling in newborn infants. Unpublished masters thesis. University of Colorado Health Sciences Center, Denver, CO.

Goosen, G. M. (1989). Concept analysis: An approach to teaching physiologic variables. *Journal of Professional Nursing, 5*(1), 31-38.

Goosen, G. M., & Bush, H. A. (1979). Adaptation: A feedback process. *Advances in Nursing Science, 1*(4), 51- 65.

Gorski, P. A. (1983). Premature infant behavioral and physiological responses to caregiving interventions in the intensive care nursery. In J. D. Call, E. Galenson, & R.L. Tyson (Eds.), *Frontiers of infant psychiatry* (pp. 256-263). New York: Basic Books.

Gunnar, M. R. (1992). Reactivity of the hypothalamic-pituitary-adrenocortical system to stressors in normal infants and children. *Pediatrics, 90*(3), 492-497.

Gunnar, M. R., Connors, J., Isensee, J., & Wall, L. (1988). Adrenocortical and behavioral distress in human newborns. *Developmental Psychobiology, 21*(4), 297-310.

Gunnar, M. R., Hertsgaard, L., Larson, M., & Rigatuso, J. (1992a). Cortisol and behavioral responses to repeated stressors in the human newborn. *Developmental Psychobiology, 24*(7), 487-505.

Gunnar, M. R., Larson, M. C., Hertsgaard, l., Harris, M. L., & Brodersen, L. (1992b). The stressfulness of separation among nine-month old infants: Effects of social context variables and infant temperament. *Child Development, 63,* 290-303.

Gunnar, M. R., Mangelsdorf, S., Larson, M., & Hertsgaard, L. (1989). Attachment, temperament, and adrenocortical activity in infancy: A study of psychoendocrine regulation. *Developmental Psychology, 25*(3), 355-363.

Guzzetta, C. E., & Forsyth, G. (1979). Nursing diagnostic pilot study: Psychophysiologic stress. *Advances in Nursing Science, 2*(1), 27-44.

Harris, J. S. (1984). Stressors and stress in critical care. *Critical Care Nurse, 4*(1), 84-97.

Hester, N. O. (1993). Pain in children. *Annual Review of Nursing Research, 11,* 105-142.

Institute of Medicine (IOM) (1981). *Report of a study: Research on stress and human health.* Washington, DC: National Academy Press.

Johnson, C. C., & Strada, M. E. (1986). Acute pain response in infants: A multidimensional description. *Pain, 24,* 373-382.

Kidder, C. (1989). Reestablishing health: Factors influencing the child's recovery in pediatric intensive care. *Journal of Pediatric Nursing, 4*(2), 96-103.

Larson, M. C., Gunnar, M. R., & Hertsgaard, L. (1991). The effects of morning naps, car trips, and maternal separation on adrenocortical activity in human infants. *Child Development, 62,* 362-372.

Levine, S., & Ursin, H. (1991). What is stress? In M. R. Brown, G. F. Koob, & C. Rivier (Eds.), *Stress: Neurobiology and neuroendocrinology* (pp. 3-21). New York: Marcel Dekker, Inc.

Lindsey, A. M., Carrieri-Kohlman, V., & Page, G. G. (1993). Stress response. In V. Carrieri-Kohlman, A. M. Lindsey, & C. M. West (Eds.), *Pathophysiological phenomena in nursing: Human responses to illness* (2nd ed., pp. 397-419). Philadelphia: W. B. Saunders Company.

Lowery, B. J. (1987). Stress research: Some theoretical and methodological issues. *Image: Journal of Nursing Scholarship, 19*(1), 42-46.

Malone, S. M., Gunnar, M. R., & Fisch, R. O. (1985). Adrenocortical and behavioral responses to limb restraint in human neonates. *Developmental Psychobiology, 18*(5), 435-446.

Merskey, H., Albe-Fessard, D. G., Bonica, J. J., Carmon, A., Dubner, R., Kerr, F. W. L., Linblom, U., Mumford, J. M., Nathan, P. W., Noodenbos, W., Pagni, C. A., Renaer, M.

J., Sternbach, R. A., & Sunderland, S. (1979). Pain terms: A list with definitions and notes on usage: Recommended by the ISAP subcommittee on taxonomy. *Pain, 6*(3), 249-252.

Mills, N. M. (1989). Pain behaviors in infants and toddlers. *Journal of Pain and Symptom Management, 4*, 184-190.

Norris, S., Campbell, L. A., & Brenkert, S. (1982). Nursing procedures and alterations in transcutaneous oxygen tension in premature infants. *Nursing Research, 31*, 300-336.

Pollack, M. M., Ruttiman, U. E., & Getson, P. R. (1988). Pediatric risk of mortality (PRISM) score. *Critical Care Medicine, 16*, 1110-1116.

Rew, L. (1986). Intuition: Concept analysis of a group phenomenon. *Advances in Nursing Science, 8*(2), 18-21.

Rhoades, R., & Pflanzer, R. (1992). *Human physiology* (2nd ed., pp. 371-529). Philadelphia: Saunders College Publishing.

Ruttiman, U. E., Albert, A., Pollack, M. M., & Glass, N. L. (1986). Dynamic assessment of severity of illness in pediatric intensive care. *Critical Care Medicine, 14*(3), 215-221.

Schmeling, D. J., & Coran, A. G. (1991). Hormonal and metabolic response to operative stress in the neonate. *Journal of Parenteral and Enteral Nutrition, 15*(2), 215-238.

Selye, H. (1946). The general adaptation syndrome and the diseases of adaptation. *The Journal of Clinical Endocrinology, 6*(2), 117-202.

Selye, H. (1993). History of the stress concept. In L. Goldberger & S. Breznitz (Eds.), *Handbook of stress: Theoretical and clinical aspects* (2nd ed., pp. 7-18). New York: The Free Press.

Solomon, S., Bird, C. E., Ling, W., Iwamiya, M., & Young, P. C. M. (1967). Formation and metabolism of steroids in the fetus and placenta. *Recent Progress in Hormone Research, 23*, 297-347.

Stidham, G., & Bugnitz, M. C. (1992). Neuroendocrine response to stress. In M. C. Rogers (Ed.), *Textbook of pediatric intensive care* (2nd ed., pp. 1476-1491).

Thompson, R. H. (1986). Where we stand: Twenty years of research on pediatric hospitalization and health care. *Children's Health Care, 14*(4), 200-210.

Ursin, H., & Olff, M. (1993). The stress response. In S. C. Stanford & P. Salmon (Eds.), *Stress: From synapse to syndrome* (pp. 4-22). London: Academic Press, Harcourt Brace & Company Publishers.

Walker, L. O., & Avant, K. (1988). *Strategies for theory construction in nursing* (2nd ed.). Norwalk, CT: Appleton & Lange.

Weiner, H. (1992). The history of the concept of stress. In H. Weiner (Ed.), *Perturbing the organism: The biology of stressful experiences* (pp. 9-27). Chicago: The University of Chicago Press.

Wilson, T., & Broome, M. E. (1989). Promoting the young child's development in the intensive care unit. *Heart & Lung, 18*, 274-279.

Wolf, A. R. (1993). Treat the babies, not their stress responses (commentary). *The Lancet, 342* (8867), 319-320.

Wolf, A. R., Eyres, R. L., Laussen, P. C., Edwards, J., Stanley, I. J., Rowe, P., & Simon, L. (1993). Effect of extradural analgesia on stress responses to abdominal surgery in infants. *British Journal of Anaesthesia, 70*(6), 654-660.

Yeh, T. S. (1992). The use of scoring systems in the pediatric ICU. *Problems in Critical Care, 3*(4), 599-615.

3

Exploring the Concept of Undocumentedness: The Meaning of a Person's Immigration Status to Nursing Care

DeAnne K. Hilfinger Messias, RN, MS

Concept development is an ongoing cycle that continues through time and occurs within a particular context, such as a discipline, cultural group, or theory (Rodgers, 1993). In nursing, concept development is considered important because it serves as the basis for our attempts to describe and explain phenomena (Walker & Avant, 1995) and is one of the stages and processes of theorizing (Meleis, 1991). Belaboring the issue of the value or relevance of "borrowed" concepts is of little use in furthering knowledge development in nursing. Any concept or phenomenon of interest to nurses, whether or not it is also of interest to other disciplines, needs to be submitted to an ongoing process of development within the context of the discipline.

The existing models of concept development have focused primarily on concept analysis, and most of the concept development work in nursing has concentrated on concept analysis. The resulting gains in new knowledge development, however, have been disproportionately small. Hupcey and colleagues (see chapter 1) critically examined the methods and procedures for concept analysis derived from Wilson's model (1963/1969), and called for expanding the methodological approaches to concept development in nursing. To ensure the vitality of concept development within knowledge development in nursing, we must look beyond concept analysis and include other processes in our research and theory-building repertoire.

Concept exploration is one of the initial processes in concept development and is particularly applicable when approaching "new" concepts. Undocumentedness, a relatively new concept within the discipline of nursing, is a case in point. With the intent of participating in the ongoing process of concept development and knowledge expansion within the discipline of nursing, in this chapter is presented the case of undocumentedness as an example of concept exploration. It is begun by situating concept exploration as part of concept development, followed by an overview of the process of concept exploration and an explanation of how the process evolved in the exploration of undocumentedness.

CONCEPT EXPLORATION AS PART OF
CONCEPT DEVELOPMENT

Definition of Concept and Exploration

Concept development is dynamic and evolutionary, and involves multiple pro-cesses. Significance, use, and application were recognized by Rodgers (1993) as distinct influences within the cycle of concept development. Meleis (1991) de-scribed a number of processes used in developing concepts: defining, differentiat-ing, delineating antecedents and consequences, modeling, analogizing, and synthe-sizing. The three strategies for systematic concept development presented by Walker and Avant (1995) were analysis, synthesis, and derivation. Most recently, Meleis (in press) distinguished concept exploration, clarification, analysis, and integration as the major processes in concept development.

The existing models of concept development have focused primarily on concept analysis. Several sets of methods and procedures for concept analysis have been derived from Wilson's model (see chapter 1). Walker and Avant (1995) also delineated procedures for concept synthesis and concept derivation. The existing models, however, do not recognize or distinguish concept exploration as a distinct process within concept development, nor do they specify methods or procedures for concept exploration as part of concept development. Schwartz-Barcott and Kim's (1993) hybrid model is an exception in the sense that it incorporates an exploratory phase, although the authors do not specifically use the term. The hybrid model presents concept development as occurring in three overlapping phases: theoretical, fieldwork, and analytic. In the model, selection is rooted in nursing practice encounters and includes a careful analysis of the context in which the concept occurs. Such characteristics highlight the exploratory nature of the initial theoretical phase of the hybrid model. The result of the theoretical phase then serves as a foundation for the fieldwork phase, aimed at refining the concept, and the analytic phase, in which the theoretical and empirical findings are integrated and interpreted.

The Process of Concept Exploration

The primary purpose of exploration is to identify and situate a concept (Table 3.1). In nursing, concept exploration involves the search for answers to various questions: What is the context in which this concept occurs? What are the possible meanings for this concept? How does this concept relate to nursing and health? Why is this concept important to nursing? What more do we need to know about this concept?

As part of knowledge development in nursing, a disciplinary perspective directs the exploration in terms of examining the relationship of the concept to health, nursing practice, and health care systems. In addition, each case of concept development involves the specific perspectives of the researchers, which should be explicated. Particularly in cases of initial concept exploration, data sources should not be limited to the nursing literature. There is no limit to the sources that may be used in concept exploration, but I recommend a broad multidisciplinary search, including the lay sources.

The process of concept exploration includes searching for existing definitions; constructing conceptual and contextualized operational definitions; analyzing the social, cultural, historical, economic, political, and/or legislative contexts of the concept; exploring possible meanings and implications; identifying characteristics, and drawing the relationship of the concept to nursing and health. Outcomes of concept exploration include the identification of existing conceptual gaps and the areas in need of further research in order to fully develop the concept for nursing.

EXPLORING THE CONCEPT OF UNDOCUMENTEDNESS: THE PROCESS

Researcher Perspective on Undocumentedness

I have approached the concept of undocumentedness as both a nurse and a feminist. Bringing a feminist perspective to concept development signifies including the

TABLE 3.1 The Process of Concept Exploration: The Example of Undocumentedness

Aims and purpose of analysis	To identify and situate the concept of undocumentedness in relation to nursing and health.
Perspective	Nursing; feminist
Selection of concept	Arose from the personal interaction of nurse/researcher with the environment and undocumented immigrants.
Data sources	Dictionaries, lay and professional literature, research
Process/procedure	Personal reflexivity; constructing definitions; examining the historical, social, political, and legislative context; exploring meanings and implications; identifying characteristics; relating the concept to nursing and health.
Outcome	Identification of the gaps in understanding the concept of undocumentedness and the areas for further research and concept development

social and historical constructions of the phenomenon, exploring the complexity and diversity of subjective experience, and questioning issues of race, class, and gender (Wuest, 1994). One of the hallmarks of feminist scholarship is researcher reflexivity (Harding, 1987). Reflexivity involves the public scrutiny of the researcher's own history and assumptions, a process necessary to locate the researcher in the same critical plane as the overt subject matter. Therefore, I begin with a reflection on how my own experience led to this exploration of undocumentedness.

Selection of the Concept

My personal encounter with undocumentedness occurred within the broader context of the current U.S. social, economic, and political scene. For nearly 25 years I lived as an immigrant in Brazil. Moving to the United States in 1993, I became a "return emigrant" and my foreign-born husband and son became immigrants. Living in California, we were highly sensitive to the various social, political, and legislative manifestations of the country's latest wave of anti-immigrant sentiment. At the time of the 1994 referendum on Proposition 187, I was engaged in research exploring the health concerns of Brazilian women employed as domestic workers in California. As I witnessed the election campaign and talked to immigrant women about their work and health, I identified undocumentedness as a phenomenon embedded in, yet distinct from, immigration. Once I had identified the phenomenon, I began to raise questions about its nature and the implications in terms of health and soon realized that I had embarked on the process of concept development. I knew, however, that I was not ready to conduct a concept analysis, as described by Walker and Avant (1995). For example, I realized that before I could refine or construct model cases I needed to explore the concept and be able to situate it within the context of nursing.

Process and Outcome of the Exploration

I found that although there is a vast interdisciplinary body of literature on immigrants, immigration, and the relationship of immigration and health, very little has been written about the phenomenon of undocumentedness. In order to understand undocumentedness as it is contextually embedded, I examined the historical, social, political, and legislative context of undocumented immigration. Rooted in dictionary definitions, as well as immigration law and lay usage, I constructed definitions for undocumentedness. Drawing on the lay and professional literature, analogous situations of undocumentedness outside the context of immigration, and research I have conducted with immigrants, I then explored the meanings and implications of the concept and examined the relationship of undocumentedness to nursing and health. The final outcome of the exploration was the identification of areas in need of further research to further ongoing development of the concept of undocumentedness in the discipline of nursing.

EXPLORING UNDOCUMENTEDNESS:
THE RESULTS

Defining Undocumentedness

Definitions for undocumentedness are not found in the nursing literature, or even in dictionaries, but conceptual and contextualized operational definitions can be constructed. A document is a tangible object, usually printed or written, which is relied upon as record or proof (McKechnie, 1983). The word comes from the Latin *documentum* which means proof, example, or lesson. *Documented* refers to a person, object, or event for which proof exists. Personal documents serve as a source of data about the individual (e.g., name, age, date and place of birth). Documents also provide evidence of status or qualifications, such as nationality, education, training, licensure, or profession. The documented individual possesses written proof which, in effect, attests to her identity, status, or qualifications. Thus, *undocumentedness* can be defined as the state of lacking a written record of proof. Persons, objects, or events with no written or printed proof are considered to be *undocumented*. In broad terms, undocumented may refer to the lack of a variety of personal documents, such as a marriage license, a work permit, or driver's license.

Situating the Concept

Undocumentedness in the Context of U.S. Immigration. In the current American context, the issue of undocumentedness is specifically embedded in the larger issue of immigration, as being an immigrant and being undocumented frequently intersect in the same individual or collective group. Earlier in U.S. history, however, undocumentedness was not an issue, because immigration documents did not exist. Visas or immigration documents were not required of persons arriving on American shores prior to the Immigration Act of 1924. Since that time, entrance into the United States has been permitted only to aliens presenting an unexpired immigrant visa conferred by a U.S. consular official. In 1924 other legislation was enacted creating the U.S. Border Patrol, and in 1929 it became a misdemeanor to enter the United States by fraudulent means (U.S. Department of Justice, 1992). Historically, these measures signaled the beginning of undocumented immigration into the United States. One of the effects of these laws was a change in the status of Mexican migrant workers, who were suddenly transformed from migrants crossing a border with impunity into criminal or illegal entrants (Mirandé, 1985).

According to United States immigration law (U.S. Department of Justice, 1992), alien refers to any person who is not a citizen or national of the United States, and immigrant is any alien granted legal permanent residence in the United States. Immigrant visas may be issued before arriving in the United States or may be acquired by persons already in the country on a temporary visa through the procedure known as *adjustment to immigrant status*. A *refugee* is a person who is not in his or her country of nationality because of persecution or a well-founded fear of persecution. Technically, a person who either enters or remains in the United States without following established immigration procedures is an *undocumented alien.*

A number of factors have contributed to the recent increase in the number of undocumented immigrants in the United States. These include: the expansion of global air transportation and the resultant difficulties for border control; the cessation of the Bracero Programs, which had provided temporary jobs for some 4 million Mexicans before 1960; the effects of the Immigration Act of 1965, which was based on a growing commitment to racial equality but which failed to directly address the issue of illegal entry and residence; and inability of intended legislation, such as the Immigration Reform and Control Act (IRCA) of 1986 and the Immigration Act of 1990, to slow the flow of undocumented immigrants into the country (Brinkley, 1994; Pear, 1995; Simon, 1995; U.S. Department of Justice, 1992). In addition, other factors, such as global economic trends, economic and political instability in other countries, and the continuing demand for low-wage, unskilled labor in the United States have also played a part in fostering the increase in the number of undocumented immigrants (Colen, 1990; Margolis, 1994).

Undocumentedness and Health in the Current Political Context. In November 1994, California voters passed a legislative proposal known as Proposition 187, with the intention of denying undocumented immigrants access to publicly funded education and health care. Although passed by 59% of the voters, Proposition 187 violated long-standing federal and state laws requiring hospitals to provide emergency care for anyone, regardless of immigration status, and the 1982 Supreme Court ruling that any child residing in the United States has the right to an education (Verhovek, 1994). Initially only the provisions relating to the manufacture, use, or sale of false immigration documents went into effect following the election, as implementation of the education, health, social services, and law enforcement provisions of the proposition was blocked temporarily by a court injunction order ("Increase in Hate Violence Follows 187," 1995). A year later, U.S. District Judge Mariana Pfaelzer ruled that portions of the measure conflict with federal power over immigration and struck down the requirements that teachers, health care workers, and social workers collect and report information about immigration status. Her ruling, however, did not preclude denial of public benefits paid for solely by the state, such as prenatal care and long-term care for the elderly (Holding, 1995). While the final outcome of Proposition 187 is being determined in the courts, other immigration reforms are under consideration in Washington. In the process, undocumented immigrants have become a significant political, economic, and health care issue.

Operationalizing and Identifying Undocumentedness

Although the United States government does not issue identification cards to citizens, it does issue identification cards to immigrants. This document, commonly known as the green card, is proof of immigration status and permission to be legally employed in the United States. Thus, in terms of U.S. immigration, the current operational definition of undocumentedness is *not possessing a valid green card.*

There are no definitive, outward characteristics of being undocumented, despite the currently widespread negative stereotype which brands Mexicans in particular and Latinos in general as potential illegal aliens. Verification that a person does not possess authentic documents is the only way to identify undocumentedness. Systematic verification of documents is not as common in the United States as it is in many other countries. For example, it is not generally required that U.S. citizens and residents carry documents with them at all times for routine presentation and inspection, attach notarized copies of social security cards to their income tax declaration, or present diplomas when applying for a job. In fact, until recently, Social Security cards contained a disclaimer that their use was only for Social Security or tax purposes, not for identification (Kuttner, 1994).

Meanings and Implications of Undocumentedness

The meaning of undocumentedness is contextually determined, but may include being illegal, illegitimate, immoral, uncounted, undercounted, unaccounted for, invisible, blamed, vulnerable, exploited, marginalized, or uninsured. Some of the possible consequences of undocumentedness include lack of legal protection; vulnerability and discrimination in the labor market; lack of social security and health care; and political, economic, ecological, social, and cultural marginalization (Velminirovic, 1979).

There is very little research concerning disclosure of undocumentedness or the perceived meaning of undocumentedness in terms of immigration, but fear has been noted to accompany undocumentedness. Colen (1990) reported the words of a West Indian woman who had worked as a live-in domestic in order to obtain her green card:

> I just wanted to know I would achieve the card. The green card was the most important thing on my mind. I wanted to get it. Because it was like I was living in fear in the country without it. When I hadn't it, I was always in fear, thinking well probably some day police could just hold me and send me back home, you know because I was illegal all that time. (p. 100)

Many of the women in Colen's study reported a sense of freedom, happiness, and thankfulness when they did obtain their legal permanent resident status. Although the meanings and implications of undocumentedness are influenced by the current political and social climate in the United States, they may vary across age, gender, ethnicity, nationality, or social class. Dunn (1995) related the story of a young undocumented immigrant from Sicily. At age 20, he arrived at Kennedy International Airport, picked up his baggage and headed for a relative's home, where he has stayed for the past 4 years. He was reported to have said, "Life is pretty normal. Everybody knows I'm illegal. It's not a big deal" (p. A5).

Legality. The notion of documentation is intricately tied to legality. In itself, the act of possessing documents often confers a legal status or a sense of legality. Conversely, the lack of documents has the effect of transforming the individual into an "illegal" or "illegitimate" person. In turn, the illegality conveys and confers a sense of immorality on the undocumented person. A woman who has a baby but lacks a marriage license becomes a mother of an illegitimate child; undocumented immigrant workers are referred to in both the lay and professional press as illegal aliens.

The authenticity of documents is another legal aspect of undocumentedness. Falsification of documents dates back to the Middle Ages. The primary focus of diplomatics, the study of documents, is to distinguish between genuine and false documents. One of the major legal ramifications of undocumentedness is the proliferation of false or forged documents used by undocumented immigrants. Current law holds employers accountable for hiring properly documented workers. In effect, an employer need only make a reasonable effort to examine a worker's documents, such as a Social Security card. In practice, such documents are widely forged, falsified, or misused (Kuttner, 1994).

Restricted Mobility and Access. Documents allow for and permit mobility; it follows that undocumentedness may impede or restrict movement. Persons who do not have documents may be detained if they are attempting to cross borders. In the same vein, apprehension of an individual's documents may also result in restriction of movement. Margolis (1994) noted that for Brazilians in New York City, "more than anything else, a green card means that its holder can enter and leave the United States at will—visit friends and relatives in Brazil, and then return to the United States unimpeded" (p. 24). In addition to restrictions on physical mobility, undocumentedness may also impede social and labor force mobility and restrict access to information, aid, and assistance (Martin, 1992).

Uncounted and Unnoticed. Being undocumented often means being uncounted (Colen, 1990). Official statistics of the Immigration and Naturalization Service (INS) do not include undocumented aliens. Although the United States census is intended to include all persons residing in the country, regardless of immigration status, undercount of undocumented immigrants is a recognized phenomenon (Margolis, 1995). Immigrant status per se is one reason for the undercount (Dauny, 1992). The undercount of undocumented immigrants is also related to language difficulties, residential mobility, living arrangements and household composition, time inaccessibility, ethnic invisibility, and fear of identification (Margolis, 1995). Unnoticed and unaccounted for, many undocumented immigrants "simply melt away into American society and bide their time until they can become legal residents" (Dunn, 1995, p. A5).

Vulnerable and Exploited. Being undocumented means being vulnerable, which may lead to exploitation by others. Although undocumentedness can affect men, women, and children, women are particularly vulnerable to exploitation because of their undocumented status. The classic analogous example is the damage and abuse suffered by women who bear children in the absence of a documented marriage. Solinger (1994) studied the racial implications of such "illegitimate" births in the United States, and noted that for both Black and White girls and women, being single and pregnant could become a weapon used by others to keep them vulnerable, defenseless, and dependent. Colen (1990) reported that some employer-sponsors of undocumented West Indian housekeepers exploited these women and manipulated their undocumented status and dependence to their advantage. The women, trapped by fears of not finding other employment and by their need of obtaining a green card, were often underpaid and overworked. Colen likened their situation to "legally sanctioned indentured servitude" (p. 89).

Undocumented immigrant workers, especially women, are often underpaid. The situation for undocumented women in agricultural wage labor (who are disproportionately Chicanas) continues to be one of extremely low wages and exploitation, in large part due to their undocumented status (Amott & Matthaei, 1991). Government sources reported that 37% of all U.S. hourly workers in private households were paid less than the minimum wage. In comparison, 44% of the legalized alien population working in private households received less than the minimum (U.S. Department of Justice, 1992).

Subject to Discrimination. An increase in discriminatory practices has been linked to the phenomenon of undocumentedness. Immigrants and American citizens of Latin American heritage, particularly Chicanos, are finding themselves increasingly subjected to intense suspicions, resentment, and in many cases, outright discrimination (Hershey, Jr., 1995). While the majority of American citizens are never required to present documents attesting to their citizenship within the borders of the United States, American citizens of Latin heritage have felt the discriminatory effect of being asked to present a social security card, or even a green card, which as citizens they do not have. In 1990 the General Accounting Office released a report charging that employer sanctions of the IRCA of 1986 had led to widespread harassment of and discrimination against Latino and Chicano workers who are routinely asked to prove their citizenship when applying for jobs or government benefits (Hershey, Jr., 1995).

Undocumentedness and the Informal Sector. Documents and documentation are part of the formal social and political structure; undocumentedness is part of the informal dimension of society, "not totally separated from the formal system, but rather linked to and shaped by it" (Laguerre, 1994, p. 2). In particular, undocumentedness often intersects with the informal economy. Even when undocumented workers are employed in the formal sector, they often obtain their jobs through informal networks (Laguerre, 1994; Messias, 1995).

The informal or underground economy includes quasi-legal or illegal activities, such as drug traffic, crime, and prostitution, as well as legal, but unregulated economic activities such as sweatshop work, which violates labor standards such as the minimum wage and job safety regulations, and other activities performed by undocumented workers outside the formal labor market (Amott & Matthaei, 1991; Margolis, 1994; Schoepfle, Perez-Lopez, & Griego, 1992). The underground economy is where the most marginalized labor force is found, including many people of color and immigrants. Undocumented immigrants work in the informal sector precisely because these are the sorts of jobs that are the "*least likely* to require immigrants to demonstrate their legal status" (Margolis, 1994, p. 21). Domestic work often occurs within the informal sector. The result is that immigrant domestic workers, and others in the underground economy, are often "doubly" undocumented, because they lack immigration papers and the work they do is undocumented because of the failure of employer and employee to meet required Social Security and income tax contributions.

Taking the Blame. Although the current level of foreign-born citizens and resident aliens is still far below the historical peak levels of 15% in 1890 and 1910, as immigration is increasing, so is public concern, fear, anger, and anti-immigrant sentiment. Much of the public discontent is focused on undocumented immigration, a growing public and congressional concern for the past 20 years (U.S. Department of Justice, 1992). Immigrants in general, and those that are undocumented in particular, are blamed for flooding the work force with unskilled, cheap labor, to the detriment of the native workers; depressing wages; and draining the government's resources. They are also accused of changing the ethnic balance of the country, and contributing to the creation of a growing uneducated underclass (Francis, 1995; Lind, 1995; Miles, 1995).

Characteristics of Undocumented Immigrants

To fully understand undocumentedness, it is important to examine the characteristics of undocumented immigrants. Despite the stereotype of the Mexican wetback, the undocumented population is actually quite diverse and heterogeneous. Undocumented immigrants come from countries as diverse as Canada, Ireland, Italy, Bahamas, Brazil, Poland, and the Philippines. Along the southern border, especially in California, Texas, and Arizona, there is a large concentration of undocumented Mexicans and Central Americans. These groups make up only a small portion of the undocumented immigrant population outside those areas, however. In New York State, the largest undocumented immigrant populations are Italians, Poles, and Ecuadorians, with Mexicans comprising just 2% of the state's undocumented population (Dunn, 1995).

Until recently, most of the undocumented immigrants arriving from Mexico were poor, male agricultural workers. Again, this stereotype does not hold for the majority of undocumented immigrants. The undocumented immigrants living in the northeastern United States are largely educated, middle- and lower-middle-class persons of urban origin, who were employed in their country of origin (Margolis,

1994). In addition to work in tomato fields and vineyards, many undocumented men find jobs in services and manufacturing, and can be found working in hotels, restaurants, night clubs, garment factories, parking garages, taxi cabs, and shoe shine stands. Others are self-employed street vendors or gardeners (Amott & Matthaei, 1991; Laguerre, 1994; Margolis, 1994).

The proportion of undocumented women is also on the rise. Despite the lack of official statistics, it is well known that a significant number of undocumented immigrant women are employed in private households as house cleaners, nannies, or baby-sitters (Amott & Matthaei, 1991; Colen, 1990; Margolis, 1994). A recent study of the population of legalized immigrants resulting from the IRCA of 1986 is an indirect indication of the level of undocumented immigrants in domestic employment (U.S. Department of Justice, 1992). This study showed that previously undocumented immigrants were seven times more likely to be household or food service workers than the general U.S. population.

Since undocumentedness often means being uncounted and unaccounted for, it is very difficult to know how many undocumented immigrants actually enter and remain in the United States. Because there are no accurate records or ways to monitor the influx of undocumented immigrants, estimates must be calculated from other sources of data, including air passenger data, census surveys, numbers of tourist visas granted, and other indirect immigration service statistics (Brinkley, 1994; Dunn, 1995; Margolis, 1994, 1995). One approximate measure of the entry of undocumented immigrants is the number of illegal aliens apprehended by the Border Patrol (Brinkley, 1994). Presumably, the number of apprehensions increases when the number of people trying to cross the border increases. Although a significant number of Mexican immigrants arrive in the United States clandestinely, however, that is not necessarily the case with undocumented immigrants from other countries. Current estimates are that less than half of the undocumented immigrants residing in the country are illegal border crossers. While border controls are focused on the Mexican border, there is relatively little deterrence for immigrant overstayers. For example, in 1994, out of 39,000 deportations, only about 600 people were deported for overstaying their visas (Dunn, 1995).

It is important to point out that undocumentedness is not necessarily a permanent characteristic or state of being; more often it is a temporary or transitory status. The majority of undocumented aliens actually arrive in the United States with valid student, business, or tourist visas. Having entered the country legally, these individuals become undocumented by overstaying their temporary visa or by working while on a visa which does not permit employment (Dunn, 1995; Margolis, 1994, 1995). On the other hand, undocumentedness is shed when the individual either leaves the country or becomes a permanent resident of the United States, either through sponsored employment, marriage, the visa lottery, or legalization sanctions such as those of the IRCA. Employer sponsorship for legal residency status is a lengthy process that often takes years from the time of first filing to obtaining the green card (Colen, 1990). The employer must obtain Department of

Labor certification that there are no documented workers available in the area to perform the same work at the prevailing wage, and the undocumented worker needs to petition the Immigration and Naturalization Service and provide evidence of at least one year of experience at similar work.

Current estimates of the number of undocumented persons residing in the United States tend to be around 4 million, although they range as high as 12 million (Amott & Matthaei, 1991; Holmes, 1995; Verhovek, 1994). An estimated 1.8 million undocumented persons live in California alone (Brinkley, 1994). Others estimate that 300,000 new immigrants enter and settle in the United States each year without the requisite documents (Bikales, 1994). But as Margolis (1994) aptly noted, such estimates are highly speculative, since "people who are in the United States illegally, of whatever nationality, are not anxious to make their presence known nor to stand up and be counted" (p. 14).

Undocumentedness and Health

Similar to the plight of other marginalized and invisible populations, the health of undocumented immigrants has not figured as a priority on many research agendas. Although relatively little is known about the health and well-being of undocumented immigrants per se, there is some evidence in the literature of the implications of undocumentedness when it comes to access to and utilization of health care. In a study of Mexican immigrants in San Diego, Chavez, Cornelius, and Jones (1985) found that both documented and undocumented respondents displayed a pattern of medical insurance coverage distinctly below that of the general U.S. population. Over 60% of the entire sample did not have private health insurance; and over 80% of the undocumented immigrants in the sample did not have medical insurance coverage. These authors proposed that the combination of low incomes and the lack of medical insurance resulted in decreased ability to afford the high cost of health care.

Weitzman and Berry (1992) have suggested, however, that insurance and income status are not in themselves sufficient explanations for differences in health care utilization among immigrants. In another study, documentation status was found to compound cultural, financial, and linguistic barriers, leading to a relatively low use of preventive health services among low-income Caribbean female immigrants (Fruchter, Remy, Burnett, & Boyce, 1986). Laguerre (1994) noted that undocumented immigrants in the San Francisco Bay area used folk medical practices extensively because they were afraid to use formal health care facilities due to their immigration status.

In a study recently conducted with Brazilian immigrants, although participants' immigration status was not asked or verified, most of the participants directly or indirectly indicated their undocumented status. The analysis of the interview data revealed various barriers to access and utilization of the U.S. health care system

(Messias, 1995). Personal barriers included expectations about provider practices, health care availability and costs, personal language skills, lack of knowledge or information, and a sense of transience. Economic and financial barriers included insurance costs and the cost of health care, measured both in terms of out-of-pocket costs and loss of income when the woman had to miss work to seek care. Fear was another barrier, stemming from the social and political climate created by the campaign and passage of Proposition 187, which occurred in the middle of the data collection process of the study. In the face of these barriers to the formal health care system, the participants either delayed seeking treatment or utilized alternative resources and providers, such as home remedies, Brazilian prescription drugs obtained locally or from Brazil, and informal providers outside the formal health care system (Messias, 1995).

The results of this study suggested that undocumented immigrants may utilize and function within informal social structures on a number of accounts, such as the use of informal health care providers and informal health care resources. Even when utilizing the formal health system, the tendency was for participants to gain access through informal networks rather than the formal referral system (Messias, 1995).

Implementation of public policies such as California's Proposition 187 would of course create even further barriers to health care. In the long term, lack of health care and medical treatment among undocumented immigrants, whether publicly mandated or not, undoubtedly will contribute to the spread of illness and disease and have negative implications for the health of undocumented immigrants in particular, as well as for that of the general public (Higbee, 1995; Katz, 1994; Lo & Ziv, 1995). For example, because treatment for tuberculosis is unlikely to be considered as requiring emergency medical care in terms of federal law, it is possible that undocumented immigrants may delay seeking care or be denied care, which could very well contribute to the resurgence of a tuberculosis epidemic (Lo & Ziv, 1995). The implications of lack of prenatal care among undocumented immigrant women are equally troubling, since lack of prenatal care is a well-known correlate of low birth weight and other perinatal and neonatal health problems.

In addition to affecting access and patterns of health care utilization, undocumentedness may also serve as a barrier to the effective establishment of a trusting relationship between health care provider and client. As is the case of other marginalized persons, a sense of vulnerability and the need for secrecy may characterize how undocumented immigrants approach encounters with nurses and other providers. In assessing clients' health status, history, behaviors, and attitudes, nurses constantly engage in processes of gathering information. Inquiries into personal history and habits may put undocumented immigrants in a position of perceived vulnerability or increase their fears of discrimination. Undocumented immigrants, like other marginalized populations, may feel compelled to use secrecy to hide personal information for self-protection and survival (Hall, Stevens, & Meleis, 1994).

FURTHERING CONCEPT DEVELOPMENT

According to Rodgers and Knafl (1993), effective concept development "should provide some release from ambiguity, enhance understanding, and provide direction for continuing development" (p. 236). In exploring the concept of undocumentedness, I have based this discussion on what is known about undocumented immigrants. The scarcity of available data has, of course, been a major limitation. In addition, the perspective of the knowledge and information that does exist is primarily of outside observers, not of undocumented persons themselves. For who dares to ask, who dares to talk, who dares to listen to the voice of the undocumented immigrant? But without hearing the voices of the undocumented themselves, we can only speculate, hypothesize, and try to imagine what the experience of undocumented immigration is actually like.

Wuest (1994) proposed that concepts must be grounded in experience and defined in ways that are meaningful for those living them. To fully develop the concept of undocumentedness, there are a number of other questions that need to be answered: What are the meanings of undocumentedness from the perspective of those who are undocumented? How does undocumentedness affect the immigration transition and how do gender, class, and ethnicity figure in this experience? In what ways is the immigration experience of the undocumented different from that of documented immigrants? How do undocumented immigrants perceive the "risk" or "costs" of being undocumented? What does disclosing their immigration status mean to undocumented aliens? What are the risks or benefits of disclosure for the client and for the health care provider? How are health beliefs, attitudes, expectations, and practices contextualized within the social, economic, and cultural realities of undocumented immigration? Various authors have advocated the use of qualitative research methods for concept development (Morse, 1995; Rodgers, 1993; Schwartz-Barcott & Kim, 1993; Walker & Avant, 1995). These methods would be particularly suited for research that would further develop the concept of undocumentedness.

Given the current political context, investigators interested in studying the lives and health of undocumented immigrants are faced with a number of challenges and potential difficulties. DeSantis (1990) conducted research among undocumented Haitian boat people in Miami. She called attention to the implications of doing field work among undocumented immigrants, noting they are a "population generally at risk for social, legal, political, and economic repercussions resulting from participation in the research or use of research results" (p. 359).

CONCLUSION

Undocumentedness refers to the lack of written proof of identity or status but has multiple meanings and implications. In the United States, the current context of undocumented immigration is an artifact of history, legislation, public policy, and economic and social contexts both locally and globally. There are multiple political, economic, social, and public health implications of undocumented status. Women are particularly vulnerable to exploitation as a result of undocumentedness. The possible meanings and implications of undocumentedness include being considered illegal, being uncounted, unnoticed, vulnerable, exploited, discriminated against, and blamed for current social and economic ills. Undocumentedness may affect mobility, employment prospects, and access to information and assistance. Undocumentedness implies exclusion from or marginalization within the formal social structure and increases the likelihood of participation in the informal sector. The existing research definitely suggests that undocumented immigrants face significant personal and structural barriers to access and utilization of the formal health care system and often rely on informal sector resources. Undocumentedness may affect relationships and information exchanges between health care providers and clients, due to clients' increased sense of vulnerability and perceived need for secrecy and self-protection.

This exploration of the concept of undocumentedness has identified and situated undocumentedness in relation to the discipline of nursing. The process of concept development needs to be carried further, however, and more research is warranted for nurses and other health care practitioners to fully understand the experience of undocumented immigrants and the implications of their immigration status for their health and well-being.

REFERENCES

Amott, T., & Matthaei, J. (1991). *Race, gender, and work: A multicultural economic history of women in the United States.* Boston: South End Press.

Bikales, G. (1994). The golden rule in the age of the global village. In N. Mills (Ed.), *Arguing immigration: The debate over the changing face of America* (pp. 199-210). New York: Touchstone.

Brinkley, J. (1994, October 15). 80's policies on illegal aliens are now haunting California: Politicians wincing after getting their wish. *The New York Times.* 1, 9.

Chavez, L. R., Cornelius, W. A., & Jones, O. W. (1985). Mexican immigrants and the utilization of U.S. health services: The case of San Diego. *Social Science and Medicine, 21*(1), 93-102.

Colen, S. (1990). "Housekeeping" for the green card: West Indian household workers, the state, and stratified reproduction in New York. In R. Sanjek & S. Colen (Eds.), *At work in homes: Household workers in world perspective* (American Ethnological Society Monograph Series, Number 3, (pp. 89-118). Washington, DC: American Anthropological Association.

Dauny, J. (1992). *The census undercount, the underground economy, and undocumented migration: The case of Dominicans in Santurce, Puerto Rico.* Washington, DC: Center for Survey Methods Research, Bureau of the Census.

DeSantis, L. (1990). Fieldwork with undocumented aliens and other populations at risk. *Western Journal of Nursing Research. 12*, 359-372.

Dunn, A. (1995, January 3). Greeted at nation's front door, many visitors stay on illegally. *New York Times.* A1, A5.

Francis, D. R. (1995, May 19). A gain-and-loss view of immigrants in U.S. *The Christian Science Monitor,* p. 20.

Fruchter, R. G., Remy, J. C., Burnett, W. S., & Boyce, J. G. (1986). Cervical cancer in immigrant Caribbean women. *American Journal of Public Health, 76,* 797-799.

Hall, J. M., Stevens, P. E., & Meleis, A. I. (1994). Marginalization: A guiding concept for valuing diversity in nursing knowledge development. *Advances in Nursing Science, 16,* 23-41.

Harding, S. (1987). *Feminism and methodology: Social science issues.* Bloomington, IN: Indiana University Press.

Hershey, Jr., R. D. (1995, April 27). Bias hits Hispanic workers: Latino labor force in the U.S. is losing ground. *The New York Times,* C1, C6.

Hessler, J. (1994). Gender-based asylum. In N. Mills (Ed.), *Arguing immigration* (pp. 211-214). New York: Touchstone.

Higbee, R. (1995). Ballot measure would endanger public health: UCSF medical ethics expert blasts Proposition 187. *Newsbreak, 10,* 1-2.

Holding, R. (1995, November 21). Prop. 187 ruled mostly illegal: Illegal-immigrant measure said to conflict with federal powers. *San Francisco Chronicle,* A1, All.

Holmes, S. A. (1995, August 30). A surge in immigration surprises experts and intensifies a debate. *The New York Times,* A1, A10.

Hondagneu-Sotelo, P. (1994). Regulating the unregulated?: Domestic workers' social networks. *Social Problems, 41*(1), 50-64.

Hupcey, J.E., Morse, J.M., Lenz, E.R., & Tasón, M.C. (1996). Wilsonian methods of concept analysis: A critique. *Scholarly Inquiry for Nursing Practice, 10*(3), 185-210.

Increase in hate violence follows 187. (1995, Spring). *CIRRS Update, 3.*

Katz, L. (1994). Jews fight initiative on illegals. *Jewish Bulletin of Northern California, 143*(26), 1, 3.

Knafl, K. A., & Deatrick, J. A. (1993). Knowledge synthesis and concept development in nursing. In B. L. Rodgers & K. A. Knafl (Eds.), *Concept development in nursing: Foundations, techniques, and applications* (pp. 35-50). Philadelphia: W. B. Saunders.

Kuttner, R. (1994). Illegal immigration: Would a national ID card help? In N. Mills (Ed.), *Arguing immigration* (pp. 81-84). New York: Touchstone.

Laguerre, M. S. (1994). *The informal city.* London: Macmillan.

Lind, M. (1995, September 7). Liberals duck immigration debate. *The New York Times,* A19.

Lo, B., & Ziv, T. A. (1995). Denial of care to illegal immigrants. *New England Journal of Medicine, 332*(16), 1095-1098.

Margolis, M. L. (1995). Brazilians and the 1990 United States Census: Immigrants, ethnicity, and the undercount. *Human Organization, 54*(1), 52-59.

Margolis, M. S. (1994). *Little Brazil: An ethnography of Brazilian immigrants in New York City.* Princeton, NJ: Princeton University Press.

Martin, S. F. (1992). *Refugee women.* London: Zed Books.

McKechnie, J. L. (1983). *Webster's New Twentieth Century Dictionary* (2nd ed.). New York: Prentice Hall.

Meleis, A. I. (1991). *Theoretical nursing: Development and progress* (2nd ed.). Philadelphia: J. B. Lippincott.

Meleis, A. I. (in press). *Theoretical nursing: Development and progress* (3rd ed.). Philadelphia: J. B. Lippincott.

Messias, D. K. H. (1995). Two lenses, one data set: Grounded theory and narrative analyses of interview with Brazilian women employed in domestic work in the Bay Area. Unpublished manuscript, University of California, San Francisco, CA.

Miles, J. (1995, April). The coming immigration debate. *The Atlantic Monthly*, 130-140

Mirandé, A. (1985). *The Chicano experience: An alternative perspective.* South Bend, IN: University of Notre Dame Press.

Morse, J. M. (1995). Exploring the theoretical basis of nursing using advanced techniques of concept analysis. *Advances in Nursing Science, 17*(3), 31-46.

Pear, R. (1995, June 5). Change in policy for immigration is urged by panel. *The New York Times.* A1, A7.

Rodgers, B. L. (1993). Concept analysis: An evolutionary view. In B. L. Rodgers & K. A. Knafl (Eds.), *Concept development in nursing: Foundations, techniques, and applications* (pp. 73-92). Philadelphia: W. B. Saunders.

Rodgers, B. L., & Knafl, K. A. (1993). Application and future directions for concept development in nursing. In B. L. Rodgers & K. A. Knafl (Eds.) *Concept development in nursing: Foundations. techniques. and applications* (pp. 235-242). Philadelphia: W. B. Saunders.

Schoepfle, G. K., Perez-Lopez, J. F., & Griego, E. (1992). The underground economy in the United States. Occasional Paper No. 2. U.S. Department of Labor.

Schwartz-Barcott, D., & Kim, H. S. (1993). An expansion and elaboration of the hybrid model of concept development. In B. L. Rodgers & K. A. Knafl (Eds.), *Concept development in nursing: Foundations, techniques, and applications* (pp. 135-257). Philadelphia: W. B. Saunders.

Simon, J. (1995, June 1). Foreign workers, American dreams. *The New York Times*, A19.

Solinger, R. (1994). Race and "Value": Black and white illegitimate babies in the U.S., 1945-1965. In V. L. Ruiz & E. C. DuBois (Eds.), *Unequal sisters: A multicultural leader in U.S. women's history* (pp. 463-478). New York: Routledge.

U.S. Department of Justice. (1991). *1990 statistical yearbook of the immigration and naturalization service.*

U.S. Department of Justice. (1992). *Immigration reform and control act: Report on the legalized alien population.*

Velminirovic, B. (1979). Forgotten people—health of the migrants. *Bulletin of the Pan American Health Organization, 13*(1), 66-85.

Verhovek, S. H. (1994, June 8). Stop benefits for aliens? It wouldn't be so easy. *The New York Times*, A1, A12.

Walker, L. O., & Avant, K. C. (1995). *Strategies for theory construction in nursing* (3rd ed.). Norwalk, CT: Appleton & Lange.

Weitzman, B. C., & Berry, C. A. (1992). Health status and health care utilization among the New York City home Attendants: An illustration of the needs of working poor, immigrant women. *Women and Health, 19*(2/3), 87-105.

Wilson, J. (1969). *Thinking with concepts.* Cambridge, England: Cambridge University Press. (Original work published in 1963)

Wuest, J. (1994). A feminist approach to concept analysis. *Western Journal of Nursing Research, 16*(5), 577-586.

Part II

Other Approaches, Future Directions

4

Choosing a Strategy for Concept Analysis in Nursing Research: Moving Beyond Wilson

Janice M. Morse, PhD (Nurs.),
PhD (Anthro.), FAAN
Judith E. Hupcey, RN, EdD
Carl Mitcham, PhD
Elizabeth R. Lenz, PhD, RN, FAAN

The abstract meanings of some of the psychosocial and behavioral concepts used in nursing research make concept analysis an important and difficult task. Psychosocial and behavioral concepts are not always about concrete, observable, and directly measurable things or phenomena and may often only be indirectly inferred. Because of the abstract nature of these concepts, their definitions are subject to considerable debate. As one comprehensive analysis of the conceptual foundations of science has argued,

> The growth and evolution of our thinking is... a process of forming concepts and of elaborating the more or less systematic structures within which these concepts are related to each other. But beyond this, once we articulate such concepts we may study these meanings and their relations themselves. That is, we may critically reflect on our understanding and study not simply what our concepts are about but the concepts themselves. (Wartofsky, 1968, p. 6)

Indeed, from this perspective, science is constituted by the movement from common sense to the conscious criticism of concepts (Wartofsky, 1968). Emerging concepts are thus tentatively introduced to the scientific community (Wallace, 1983), and as they are criticized and gain acceptance through the

Acknowledgment. The assistance of Dr. M. Cerdas Tasón is acknowledged. This research is supported by NIH, NINR, 2R01 NR02130-07 (J. M. Morse) and AHCPR, F32 H500094-02 (J. E. Hupcey).

development of a critical consensus, the understanding of the concepts increases; as research develops, the definitions of concepts evolve and eventually stabilize.

The result is that during a period of the introduction or critical assessment of concepts—what Thomas Kuhn (1970) might call a pre-paradigmatic phase in scientific development—similar theoretical explanations often compete for preferred acceptance, while allied concepts vie to account for the same phenomenon. Alternatively, one concept may have several definitions; and in some cases these various meanings may be implicit, unrecognized by researchers and clinicians, resulting in a lack of clarity that makes nursing a soft science—or at least softer than is desirable (for example, consider the case of caring [Morse, Bottorff et al., 1992]). Thus, the utilization of poorly understood concepts in research will, at the most basic level, result in questionable reliability and validity in excessive and antagonistic discourse between researchers, and in misunderstanding in the communication of research findings to both the scientific community and to practitioners.

Nevertheless, despite a recognized need for *concept analysis* in nursing research, as reflected by the increasing numbers of articles on this topic in nursing journals, the majority of articles are simplistic, describing or defining the attributes of a concept in a manner that adds little to nursing knowledge. In some of these articles the resulting attributes are so vague and general that they may even just as well be applied to another concept (Morse, 1995). In the first chapter we have argued that the Wilsonian methods, on which the majority of concept analyses in nursing are based, have been simplified and have been inappropriately adopted and adapted. In addition, the bulk of the responsibility for concept analysis has been assigned to graduate students, with publications arising from their class assignments (Morse, in review). Partitioning such an important task to our most inexperienced researchers undermines the significance of this endeavor. In this chapter, we will evaluate the approaches and methods used in concept analysis in nursing research and argue that methodological development for enhancing concept analysis is urgently required. We will limit discussion in this chapter to psychosocial and behavioral concepts, which are defined as stable organizations of experiences of reality, achieved through the utilization of rules of relation, and to which a name has been given (Bolton, 1977). Briefly, Bolton's rules of relation are expressions of the ways an experience is organized according to intention; the results of particular instances become general according to rules that are stabilized in language and are the results of coordination. Individuals use concepts to organize events, to identify future events or instances, and to make sense between acts and related stimulus conditions (Bolton, 1977; see also Morse, 1995). In summary, the kinds of concepts with which we are most concerned have the following characteristics: They are abstract, and the meaning of the concept cannot be directly observed but must be identified by its indicators and examined by inference using Bolton's rules of relation. Furthermore, as such concepts mature through critical assessment, there is increasing consensus as to their meanings, and the meanings become more stable. Finally, although such concepts may be manifest in various forms in different contexts, their attributes or characteristics remain recognizable.

Ideally, a mature concept should be well defined, with characteristics or attributes identified, boundaries demarcated, preconditions specified, and outcomes described (Morse, Mitcham, Hupcey, & Tasón, 1996). Once a concept is so defined, examples may easily and reliably be identified in the clinical setting. Phenomena that *are* and *are not* related to the concept are evident. A clear definition and description of the characteristics of the concept facilitates the operationalization and ultimately the identification of those variables relevant for measurement. In reality, however, all characteristics relevant to a concept may not be equally well recognized as such or equally well related. Some clinical events may be more or less poor examples of some conceptualized phenomena and, while exhibiting all the necessary characteristics, also exhibit others as well. Thus, when conducting concept analysis, the task is facilitated by the selection of clear examples or prototypes representing the concept.

Concept analysis as used in this chapter refers to a process of inquiry that explores concepts for their level of development or maturity as revealed by their internal structure, use, representativeness, and/or relations to other concepts. Concept analysis entails an assessment process using various techniques to explore the description of a concept in the literature or to develop a concept from observational and/or interview data. Thus, concept analysis is a term referring to the process of unfolding, exploring, and understanding concepts for the purposes of concept development, delineation, comparison, clarification, correction, identification, refinement, and validation. For us, concept analysis is a broad term that encompasses numerous kinds of concept-related activities. We are aware, however, that this terminology differs from that used by other nurse authors (e.g., Walker & Avant) who use "concept development" as the most encompassing term and "concept analysis" as a more specific activity. The research strategy used depends on the purpose of inquiry and on the level of maturity of a concept.

In this chapter, we will explore the state of concept analysis in nursing research by describing and critiquing the four most generally adopted methods: (1) Wilsonian (1963/1969) methods of concept analysis, that is those adopted by Walker and Avant (1983/1988/1995) and Chinn and Jacobs (1983/1987) and Chinn and Kramer (1991) and further modified by Schwartz-Barcott and Kim (1986/1993) and Rodgers (1989/1993), (2) qualitative methods for concept analysis, (3) critical analysis of a concept using the literature as data, and (4) quantitative methods for concept analysis. Prior to this critical assessment, however, we provide a background on concept analysis outside nursing and some general remarks on the use of concepts in nursing. Afterward, by way of conclusion, methods for determining the appropriate approach to concept analysis research and criteria for assessing concept analysis research itself will be proposed.

EVALUATING A CONCEPT

Ideally, concepts used in a discipline should be "mature. " That is, they should be relatively stable, clearly defined, with well described characteristics, demarcated boundaries, specified preconditions and outcomes. Insofar as they have practical as well as purely cognitive meaning, they should also bear upon clinical phenomena. Bolton (1977) adds additional criteria: not only should a concept be related to present instances of a phenomenon, it should also be capable of being related to "fresh instances"—that is, to new situations, to new settings, and to new circumstances in which the phenomenon appears.

Not all concepts exhibit the same level of maturity. Because knowledge is continually developing, new concepts are being introduced, and accepted concepts continually being investigated and refined, concepts exist at various levels of development. Some concepts are poorly defined with characteristics that have not been described, related preconditions and outcomes that are unspecified and that lack demarcation. Other concepts may be consistently defined, yet when analyzed, inconsistency between the definition and its utilization in research are revealed, so that the concept is not as mature as first thought. In these and other cases, concept analysis is required to move a concept toward maturity.

Concept analysis techniques may be used to evaluate the level of maturity or the level of development of selected nursing concepts in five ways: (a) to identify gaps in nursing knowledge; (b) to determine the need to refine or clarify a concept when the concept appears sloppy or appears to have multiple meanings; (c) to evaluate the adequacy of competing concepts in their relations to phenomena; (d) to examine the congruence between the definition of the concept and the way it has been operationalized; or (e) to ascertain the fit between the definition of the concept and its clinical application.

Reviewing and summarizing the aims of concept analysis as they are developed in epistemological, logical, and linguistic philosophy, one may venture to identify the following somewhat overlapping principles:

- Concepts should be clear and distinct, that is, clearly defined and well differentiated from other concepts (epistemological principle).
- Concepts should be coherently and systematically related to other concepts (logical principle).
- Concepts should be applicable to the world or operationalized (the pragmatic principle).
- Concepts should be appropriate to their use in context (linguistic principle).

The set of criteria proposed in Morse, Mitcham, Hupcey, and Tasón (1996) can be interpreted as attempts to operationalize these principles for the context of nursing research. At the same time, one way of interpreting the state of concept analysis in nursing research is in terms of its failures or attempts to achieve one or more of these aims.

A large number of articles analyzing concepts have been published, and these have addressed concepts critical to nursing inquiry. (See Table 4.1 for example.) While many of these concepts were initially created in other disciplines and then transferred into nursing (e.g., social support, empathy, hardiness, etc.), only one has emerged directly from nursing (e.g., compathy). The range of topics is critical to the foundation of nursing science, nursing theory and nursing research.

Despite the importance of developing concepts and the relative frequency that articles on concept analysis are published, the actual description of the methods used to explore and analyze concepts has, until recently, not been explicitly examined or critiqued. Table 4.1 presents examples of concept analysis in nursing describing the methods used for each. The remainder of this chapter will critique these methods.

ADEQUACY OF METHODS FOR DEVELOPING CONCEPTS

Wilson-Derived Methods

As discussed in chapter 1, the most frequently used method for concept analysis in nursing is based on the approach developed by Wilson (1963/1969). It was adapted into nursing during the early 1980s as a step in the process of nursing theory development. In 1983, Walker and Avant and Chinn and Jacobs used Wilson's techniques as a basis for their methods of concept analysis. As adopted, this method of concept analysis typically involved an 8-step technique: (a) select a concept; (b) determine the aims or purpose of analysis; (c) determine the defining attributes; (d) construct a model case; (e) construct borderline, related, contrary invented, and illegitimate cases; (f) identify antecedents and consequences; and (g) define empirical referents (Walker & Avant, 1988). Modifications of these techniques were subsequently adapted and introduced by Rodgers (1993) and Schwartz-Barcott and Kim (1986, 1993). (Problems with these techniques as described by Hupcey and colleagues in chapter 1 will be briefly summarized in what follows.)

One problem with the adaptation of Wilson's method is that these derivations lack the intellectual rigor required by Wilson. The major positive aspect of Walker and Avant's adaptation is that it appears to be a set of easily followed steps. However, this is also a major flaw: this "ease" has led many nurse researchers to believe that concept analysis is a simple procedure and, by following 8 steps, significant results will be obtained. Furthermore, Wilson-derived methods stress only the linguistic principle at the expense of the epistemological, logical, and pragmatic principles discussed earlier.

Schwartz-Barcott and Kim's (1986, 1993) hybrid model was specifically designed as a graduate student assignment and as a method that would improve

TABLE 4.1 Topics of Concept Analysis by Method (1980-Present)

Wilsonian Methods	Qualitative Analysis	Analysis of the Literature	Quantitative Analysis[1]
Wilson (Walker & Avant)	Benevolence [grounded theory] (Lützen & Nordin, 1993)	Caring (Morse, Solberg, Neander et al., 1990)	Belonging (Hagerty & Patusky, 1995)
Belonging (Hagerty, Lynch-Sauer, Patusky et al., 1992)	Compathy (Morse, 1994)	Caring (Morse, Bottorff, Neander & Solberg, 1991)	Empathy (La Monica, 1981)
Chronic sorrow (Lindgren, Burke, Hainsworth et al., 1992)	Health [ethnography] (Morse, 1987)	Chronic sorrow (Teel, 1991)	Hardiness (Jennings & Staggers, 1994)
Crisis (Geissler, 1984)	Hope [grounded theory] (Owen, 1989)	Comfort (Kolcaba, 1991)	Hope (Miller & Powers, 1988)
Decision making (Matteson & Hawkins, 1990)	Hope [interview data] (Morse & Doberneck, 1995)	Comfort (Kolcaba & Kolcaba, 1991)	Learned helplessness (Quinless & Nelson, 1988)
Dignity (Mairis, 1994)	Privacy [ethnography] (Applegate & Morse, 1994)	Comfort (Kolcaba, 1992)	Loneliness (Mahon & Yarcheski, 1988)
Empowerment (Hawks, 1992)	Suffering and enduring (Morse & Carter, 1996)	Coping (Panzarine, 1985)	Maternal role competence (Mercer & Ferketich, 1994)
Experience (Watson, 1991)	Touch (Estabrooks, 1989; Estabrooks & Morse, 1992)	Empathy (Morse, Anderson, Bottorff et al., 1992)	Quality of life (Ferrans & Powers, 1992)
Expert (Jasper, 1994)		Empathy (Morse, Bottorff, Anderson et al., 1992)	Social support (Norbeck, Lindsey, Carrieri, 1983)
Feminism (Allan, 1993)		Gaze (Ashmore & Ramsamy, 1993)	Uncertainty (Mishel, 1984)
Friendship (Caroline, 1993)		Health (Payne, 1983)	
Health (Simmons, 1989)		Holism (Sarkis & Skoner, 1987)	
Hope (Stephenson, 1991)		Locus of control (Arakelian, 1980)	
Hopelessness (Campbell, 1987)			
Intuition (Rew, 1986)			
Rodgers Evolutionary Method			
Grief (Cowles & Rodgers, 1991)			
Grief (Rodgers & Cowles, 1991)			
Health policy (Rodgers, 1989)			
Integration (Westra & Rodgers, 1991)			
Mentoring (Yoder, 1990)			
Schwartz-Barcott & Kim Hybrid			
Chronic sorrow (Phillips, 1991)			
Therapeutic alliance (Madden, 1990)			
Withdrawal (Verhulst & Schwartz-Barcott, 1993)			
Chinn & Jacobs			
Intimacy (Timmerman, 1991)			
Social isolation (Warren, 1993)			

(Continued)

TABLE 4.1 (Continued)

Wilsonian Methods	Qualitative Analysis	Analysis of the Literature	Quantitative Analysis[1]
Mother-daughter identification (Boyd, 1985)		Marginalization (Hall, Stevens, & Meleis, 1994)	
Power (Hawks, 1991)		Mastery (Younger, 1991)	
Quality of life (Meeberg, 1993)		Milieu therapy (Tuck & Keels, 1992)	
Wilson (Walker & Avant)		Nursing art (Johnson, 1994)	
Reassurance (Teasdale, 1989)		Nursing disclosure (Trandel-Korenchuk, 1986)	
Self-neglect (Reed & Leonard, 1989)		Nursing insight (Morse, et al., 1994)	
Self-nurturing (Nemcek, 1987)		Pattern (Crawford, 1982)	
Serenity (Roberts & Fitzgerald, 1991)		Privacy (Rawnsley, 1980)	
Spiritual perspective, hope, acceptance (Haase, Britt, Coward, et al., 1992)		Quality (Frost, 1992)	
Trust (Meize-Grochowski, 1984)			

[1]Examples cited in quantitative methods may not be reflected in a single source but rather in a pragmatic sequential development of the concept.

on Wilson's. The hybrid model contains many qualities that are lacking in the earlier methods, including an extensive literature review, cases that are developed from actual nursing or patient situations, some techniques of qualitative analysis, and the intellectual rigor and the working back and forth between steps (as suggested by Wilson). This method, however, utilized only one nursing situation from which only a few cases are actually examined. While this method may be appropriate as a classroom demonstration, it has limited use for the advancement of nursing knowledge, as the model lacks rigor, an adequate data base, generalizability, and utility.

Rodgers's (1993) evolutionary method places great emphasis on the selection of the literature to be reviewed, although she fails to stress the temporal comparison or intellectual rigor that is integral to Wilson. In a kind of overemphasis of the linguistic principle, Rodgers also considers concepts to be context-bound, so that the usefulness of the analysis is again restricted to a single situation. Since the evolutionary method requires that only one case representing the concept be developed, there is a loss of richness that would otherwise be obtainable with the quantity of data collected. Thus, while this method compensates for some limitations in previous developments, it remains of limited utility for nursing science.

Despite such limitations, these methods of concept analysis have been widely used to explore a vast number of concepts (see Table 4.1). Unfortunately, and perhaps due to the limitations in the methods, this work has failed to produce concomitant gains in nursing knowledge. In chapter 1 we have suggested that these articles frequently lack substance and evidence of intellectual investment. They also lack cohesion and integration, so that each step of the process is not integrated with the next or, sometimes, even with the concept under investigation. Often the conclusions are not summarized and do not enlighten the reader as to what knowledge was gained from the particular concept analysis activity.

Analysis of Qualitative Methods for Concept Analysis

Qualitative methods differ markedly from the above approaches in that they require the collection of data from participants and inductive analysis of those data. The primary purposes of qualitative methods are to organize and consolidate textual and observational data into categories, to identify the characteristics along with the antecedents and consequences of the characteristics, and to compare data so that conceptual boundaries may be identified. Comparison of one category with another enables the identification of inclusion/exclusion criteria for each concept, and this process facilitates the identification of boundaries. Techniques of synthesis and abstraction enable the description of the concept in precise analytical terms. Synthesis and abstraction are essential to lift the analysis beyond a mere description of an experience toward true conceptualization.

The selection of which qualitative method to use depends in part on the purpose of conceptual inquiry. Phenomenological methods are well suited for concept identification and concept analysis. For example, the concept of compathy (Morse, 1995) was identified when interview data did not fit into the category describing empathy. Van Manen (1991) used phenomenology to develop the concept of tact in teaching. He identified the characteristics ("How tact is manifest"), the consequences ("What does tact do?"), and the conditions ("aspects") in which it is manifested. Ethnography has also been used for concept analysis. In a study on privacy (Applegate & Morse, 1994), ethnographic data collected in a nursing home were explored to see when privacy violations occurred by moving the conceptual scheme of privacy (obtained from the literature) as a "template" over these data. This procedure enabled the investigators to identify the interpersonal conditions in which privacy violations occurred, thus developing knowledge of the concept.

The purpose of ethnoscience, to elicit cognitive categories and to develop concepts from the perspective of an informant, makes it perhaps an optimal method for concept analysis. It certainly entails, in a more balanced way than Wilson-derived methods, the utilization of what have been called the epistemological, pragmatic, and linguistic principles. Its only shortcoming is in relation to the logical principle. Unstructured interviews are analyzed to identify the concepts of significance. The characteristics of these concepts are identified using semantic techniques (such as sentence completion). The boundaries are identified using q-sorts or card sorts.

The ability of grounded theory methods to document process and changes over time, to link categories and to develop models, makes this method particularly useful for exploring categories. Examination of qualitative research that explores concepts reveals that the antecedents, consequences, and attributes are easily identified. In particular, techniques of grounded theory permit the evolving nature of the concepts to be explored. The identification of negative cases and the comparison of different contexts or populations also permit different forms of the concept to be identified and a complete description of the attributes to be obtained. The richness of qualitative data enables relationships to be diagrammed.

Finally, the combination of two qualitative techniques may be used to obtain the most comprehensive picture of the phenomenon. For instance, Estabrooks (1989) used ethnoscience as well as grounded theory in her study delineating the perception of touch. The ethnoscience provided information about the types of touch and the components of touch; grounded theory linked the characteristics together, and the antecedents and consequences completed the model.

While qualitative methods are usually used as a packaged set, complete with epistemological underpinnings and a consistent and cohesive "formula" or set of particular methods, they also may be perceived as consisting of techniques usable relatively independently of their paradigms and separately from any originally intended purposes. When viewed in this light—as a series of techniques by which data may be sorted, categories developed, and the characteristics of those categories delineated and refined—the full utility of qualitative methods for concept analysis becomes apparent. For example, the theoretical foundations of the ethnographic method (and types of ethnography, such as ethnoscience) are based on the concept of culture (i. e., the sharing of values and beliefs between members of the same culture to form a cultural reality or shared emic perspective that may be elicited through the analysis of a text). Without violating the assumptions of culture, however, one may use ethnographic techniques, such as participant observations and unstructured interviews (to techniques of ethnoscience, such as card sorts to construct a taxonomy), to understand shared concepts.

Table 4.2 provides examples of techniques from various qualitative methods that may be useful in concept analysis. The list is not comprehensive and is intended only to illustrate the applicability of various qualitative techniques for concept analysis.

The use of qualitative methods for the specific purpose of analyzing concepts is not without difficulties. When purposively seeking information about a concept in the naturalistic setting, it is easy to fall into the trap of working deductively (instead of inductively), and it requires a skilled researcher to avoid such a pitfall. Despite this problem, many researchers have used qualitative methods to explore various concepts, and these are listed by topic in Table 4.1.

Critical Analysis of the Literature for Concept Analysis

In contrast to methods derived from Wilson and to qualitative methods, the analysis of concepts based on a literature review does not have clearly defined methodological guidelines. Indeed, literature review articles often do not even include a clearly explicated method, although this lack of rigorous guidelines does not necessarily detract from usefulness. One unwritten rule—but one that is obvious—is that all such articles have selected concepts for which there is a relatively large "data base"; that is, detailed and complete descriptions exist in the literature or, alternatively, a large body of literature exists and is available for analysis. Thus, the main limitation of Wilson-derived methods, that of data inadequacy, is not an issue.

The studies that have critically analyzed a published literature as a means to concept analysis are included in Table 4.1. Interestingly, the purposes of the research cited by the researchers differ markedly from the purposes of those who have used Wilson-derived methods. Whereas those who have used Wilson-derived methods have conducted their analyses primarily for concept clarification, those who have done literature reviews exhibit more varied and complex agendas. Table 4.3 shows detailed purposes and outcomes of such research. In this case, concept analysis has usually been conducted to forward a research program or facilitate a broader research purpose rather than to conduct concept analysis for its own sake. For instance, researchers have cited concept clarification, operationalization, developing conceptual frameworks, and evaluation of the adequacy of the concept for practice as outcomes.

Although researchers are not often explicit about the techniques that they use when critically analyzing a body of literature, their techniques actually often resemble the kind of content analysis used in qualitative methods, but perhaps with more stress on what was referred to above as the logical principle. Researchers sort all content for the entire data set into categories and often form subcategories. The commonalties and differences of each category are noted and then compared with other parts of the data set so that assumptions, values, and the content may be made explicit. In addition, when comparing several allied concepts, questions are asked of the literature that address each concept, and this process facilitates the identification of comparison between the categories and subcategories for each concept (see Morse, Miles, Clark & Doberneck, 1994), thus permitting concept delineation.

TABLE 4.2 Qualitative Analytic Techniques That Facilitate Concept Analysis and Development

Qualitative Method	Techniques	Application for Concept Development
Phenomenology	Conversations	Concept identification
	Bracketing	Enables inductive development of concept
	Thematic development	Identification of conceptual characteristics
Ethnography	Unstructured interviews	Description of concepts from experience
	Participant observation	Detailed description of behaviors
Ethnoscience	Card sorts	Identification of characteristics of concept
		Identification of boundaries
	Construction of a taxonomy	Discerning relationship between characteristics
Grounded Theory	Unstructured interviews	Identification of antecedents and consequences
	Constant comparison	Identification of conceptual boundaries

TABLE 4.3 Summary of Articles Using the Literature for Concept Analysis

Concept/Author	Methods	Outcome
Caring (Morse, Bottorff et al., 1991)	Analyzed literature	Compared the five conceptualizations of caring and the development of the concepts for clinical practice
Caring (Morse, Solberg et al., 1990)	Analyzed literature	Elucidated various concepts describing the phenomena and implications for clinical practice
Chronic sorrow (Teel, 1991)	Analyzed literature—included models of grief	Identified limitations in current models, recommended implications for clinical practice and research
Comfort (Kolcaba & Kolcaba, 1991)	Analyzed literature—definitions, nursing, theories, and patient needs	Operationalized concept
Comfort (Kolcaba, 1992)	Built on the taxonomic structure of comfort (1991)	Developed a framework for organizing nursing practice
Coping (Panzarine, 1985)	Analyzed literature—evaluated research results	Recommended consideration of all conceptual dimensions for nursing research
Disclosure (Trandel-Korenchuk, 1986)	Analyzed literature—primarily moral and legal theories and contexts	Delineated characteristics and dimensions of concepts in various contexts
Empathy (Morse, Anderson et al., 1992)	Analyzed literature and compared with clinical data	Compared concept with phenomenon
Empathy (Morse, Bottorff et al., 1992)	Analyzed literature—instruments and clinical application	Evaluated conceptual fit of concept for nursing context
Gaze (Ashmore & Ramsamy, 1993)	Analyzed literature—included development, utilization or purpose of concept	Identified two conceptualizations of concepts and the fit/application to the clinical setting

(Continued)

TABLE 4.3 (Continued)

Concept/Author	Methods	Outcome
Health (Payne, 1983)	Analyzed literature—development of definitions, concepts, and models	Revised definition of health
Holism (Sarkis & Skoner, 1991)	Analyzed literature	Identified competing conceptualizations of concept
*Locus of control (Morse, Bottorff et al., 1992)	Analyzed literature—included research results	Evaluated concept and compared fit to nursing practice
Marginalization (Hall, Stevens, Meleis, 1994)	Analyzed literature/definition of related concepts	Clarified relationship of concepts and relationship to other concepts and relevance to health
Mastery (Younger, 1991)	Analyzed literature	Identified and described elements of concept and explained theoretical relationships as a theoretical basis for instrument development
Milieu therapy (Tuck & Keels, 1992)	Analyzed literature—development of concept and use in clinical practice	Recommended utilization of the concept in the clinical setting
Nursing art (Johnson, 1994)	Critical examinations and analysis—nursing literature	Understanding the structure and conceptualizations regarding nursing art
Pattern (Crawford, 1982)	Analyzed definitions of patterns by other nurses	Recommendation for nursing students based on an evaluation
Privacy (Rawnsley, 1980)	Analyzed literature—development of definitions by discipline	Clarified dimensions of concept
Quality (Frost, 1992)	Analyzed definition in literature	Implication for nursing theory practice, and research

*Presents criteria for evaluation.

Quantitative Methods for Concept Analysis

Quantitative approaches to concept analysis are generally brought into play only after considerable preliminary work has been done to generate and clarify a conceptualization. The preliminary activity may include any or all of the three methods described above to move a concept toward maturity. Once the researcher has clearly described internal characteristics of the concept and provided a well-developed theoretical definition, the next step is the use of quantitative methods to validate and refine the concept with a strong emphasis on the epistemological and pragmatic principles. The major quantitative techniques used, along with their purposes, are listed in Table 4.4.

The use of quantitative methods in concept analysis has occurred largely in conjunction with measurement. Quantitative methods generally build upon theory derived from the literature or are preceded by concept analysis using one of the other two methods. Prior to beginning a concept-based approach to measurement, a researcher needs to evaluate the original concept analysis to ensure that this step has been performed adequately. The characteristics, components and variable dimensions must be clearly defined and described (Waltz, Strickland, & Lenz, 1991); in other words, the concept must appear mature. The formation of the concept (including theoretical definitions, subdimensions, characteristics, boundaries, preconditions, and outcomes) becomes a blueprint for designing or selecting measures. Often a "conceptual mapping" (Batey, 1977) is produced in the form of a model, a set of dimensions, or a full-blown theory and then subjected to deductive quantitative testing.

Once an instrument has been developed to measure a given concept, quantitative methods are used for assessing its psychometric properties. This assessment is guided by, and the results interpreted in relation to, a given conceptualization of the phenomena in question; the results, in turn, may validate or suggest a need for refinement of the original conceptualization. For example, the most common psychometric assessment reported in the nursing literature is Cronbach's alpha, used to assess internal consistency reliability (i. e., the degree to which the items of a given scale or subscale vary together, as would be expected if they were all indicators of the same concept or aspect thereof and if respondents were consistent in their responses). It is reasonable to expect an instrument to display internal consistency reliability only if the concept being measured is unidimensional. If the conceptualization includes multiple dimensions or components that are relatively independent of one another, internal consistency reliability would be expected within subscales but not for an overall measure.

Factor analysis is being used increasingly in assessing construct validity, specifically to explore the dimensionality of the concept and the structure of its meaning. An example of this approach is Mishel's (Mishel, 1981, 1983, 1984;

Mishel & Braden, 1988; Mishel, Padilla, Grant, & Sorenson, 1991) use of factor analysis to determine the structure of the concept of uncertainty in illness.

Quantitative methods can make considerable contribution to the testing and refinement of concepts. For instance, a stringent approach to testing the structure of a given concept (i. e., the extent to which several indicators actually measure it, as opposed to another concept) is to subject it to a multiple-indicator structural equation model testing using LISREL (e.g., see Ratner, Bottorff, Johnson, & Hayduk, in press). Such analyses may reveal that a measurement model based on the theoretical conceptualization does not fit the data, thus calling the original conceptualization into question (as with Pender's model [Johnson, Ratner, Bottorff, & Hayduk, 1993]). Thus, the use of LISREL may

TABLE 4.4 Use of Quantitative Methods for Concept Analysis

Quantitative Method	Techniques	Application for Concept Analysis
Instrument Development and Testing	Factor analysis	Identification of characteristics and dimensions; Delimitation of conceptual boundaries and subconcepts
	Chronbach's Alpha	Internal consistency Assess dimensionality of subscales and total instrument
	Correlation	Determination of overlap with alternative conceptualization and related concepts
Determine causality	Regression analysis	Identification of antecedents and consequences may be used to differentiate effects of related concepts
Validation	*LISREL*	Identification of conceptual boundaries Validation of conceptualization and measurement indicators Refinement/verification of the conceptual models
	Discriminant analysis	Delineates two concepts by inclusion/exclusion

reveal the suggested configuration of indicators which may or may not make sense theoretically, so its implications need to be examined carefully.

Examples of major quantitative studies used in nursing for concept analysis are presented in Table 4.1. However, it is important to note that refinement of concepts using quantitative methods has largely been conducted with a series of studies related to measurement and instrument development. This work is not generally published as one article, but additions and revisions have been published as the instrument is refined over time.

SELECTING AN APPROACH FOR CONCEPT ANALYSIS RESEARCH

The first step in selecting an appropriate approach to concept analysis research is to determine the level of maturity of a concept. As concepts emerge, they may be poorly defined (a failure with regard to the epistemological principle). One indicator that a concept is immature is an absence of information about the concept—or allied concepts—in the literature. In particular, a lack of competing concepts may even indicate that the concept bears on a field of experience to which little attention has been devoted (a pragmatic principle issue). With little information available, one cannot identify the conceptual boundaries or parameters to recognize what questions would be relevant to ask about the concept. Attempts to compare the concept with other concepts may reveal confusion in terminology so that concepts appear to be illogical or to overlap (a failure to meet the logical principle). In such cases, investigators are advised to use qualitative methods for concept analysis. The concept will need considerable development and clarification (see Table 4.5).

By contrast, when the phenomenon is well described and internal characteristics delineated, and a concept appears mature, quantitative methods of inquiry are appropriate to "fine tune" the concept. In the case of mature concepts, there will be few if any competing concepts; the conceptual boundaries will be clearly defined, and the concept will be operationalized (see Table 4.5).

Between the two extremes of immature and mature concepts are concepts that are partially developed. Such concepts may appear to be well established and described, although some degree of conceptual confusion continues to exist, with several concepts competing to describe the same phenomenon. In such cases, it may not be necessary to collect data, but only to critically analyze the literature to further develop the concept.

Despite this, an additional consideration when selecting a method is to determine the purpose of the concept inquiry. Is it for purposes of concept development, identification, delineation, comparison, clarification, correction, or refinement and measurement? Knowledge base requirements and indicators for each of these tasks are shown in Table 4.6.

EVALUATION OF CONCEPT
ANALYSIS RESEARCH

How does one evaluate completed concept analysis research? The criteria presented in Table 4.7 are intended to guide such evaluation. These criteria are not intended as "all or nothing" evaluative tools. Instead, an evaluator should wisely weigh each criterion to determine the worthiness of the research.

TABLE 4.5 Indicators for Selecting the Optimal Research Approach

	Criteria for Assessing Level of Maturity of Concept		
Purpose	Immature	Partially Developed	Mature
1. Nature of phenomenon development	Poorly developed, poorly understood, poorly explained	Must be established and well-described	Must be well described, and internal characteristics delineated
2. Competing explanatory concepts	Gap in knowledge	Easily identified Lots of literature available describing each concept	Preferably there should be no competing concepts
3. Identify parameters and comparative questions	Difficult to identify and develop	Parameters defined Comprehensive comparative questions may be identified	Parameters clearly defined Comparative questions not relevant
4. Comparison concept(s)	Confusing, illogical or concepts overlap	May be systematically compared and differentiated using quesions	Not pertinent
5. Evaluation of analysis for concept's fit with the phenomenon	Not convincing	Comprehensive Evident	Evident: Concept should be operationalized
Research Approach (purpose)	Qualitative methods (for concept identification, development, delineation, and correction)	Critical analysis of the literature (for concept comparison, clarification, and correction) Quantitative methods (for concept exploration)	Quantitative methods (for concept validation, refinement, and measurement)

First and foremost, concept analysis demands an adequate data base. Concept analysis, whether using qualitative methods, critical analysis of the literature, or quantitative methods, must be based on rich and comprehensive data. If it is a critical analysis of the literature, then there must be ample literature—adequate to provide substance to the inquiry. If qualitative methods

TABLE 4.6 Indicators for Data Sources, and Type of Concept Analysis Inquiry

Indicators	Type of Concept Analysis Research
Multiple indices, borderline concepts exist, yet no concept accurately accounts for data describing a phenomenon[1]	Concept identification
A concept is immature, in that, while defined, the definitions may be inadequate. Descriptive information is missing regarding the characteristics, antecedents or consequences[2]	Concept development
Two concepts appear almost uniformly linked together, as if they were a part of the same experience[3]	Concept delineation
The area of inquiry is undeveloped and numerous concepts exist to explain the phenomenon and provide competing explanations[4]	Concept comparison
The concept appears "mature," and there is a large body of literature that includes definitions and rich descriptions, such as clinical exemplars and quantitative instruments, but the concept is measured using various variables and is applied in different ways in research[5]	Concept clarification
The concept appears well-developed and is defined consistently, but the application to practice appears inappropriate[6] or appears inaccurate[7]	Concept correction
The concept appears well developed, its dimensions and boundaries and potential indicators have been identified. The validity of the conceptualization across populations and contexts has not been determined.[8]	Concept refinement/ measurement

[1] e.g., compathy (Morse, 1995); [2] e.g., hope (Morse & Doberneck, 1995); [3] e.g., enduring and suffering (Morse & Carter, 1996); [4] e.g., "sensing patient needs" (Morse, Miles, Clark, & Doberneck, 1994); [5] e.g., caring (Morse, Solberg, Neander, Bottorff, & Johnson, 1990); [6] e.g., empathy (Morse, Anderson, Bottorff, Yonge, O'Brien, Solberg, & McIlveen, 1992); [7] e.g., social support (Hupcey & Morse, 1995); [8] e.g., quality of life (Ferrans & Powers, 1992).

are used, then description must be what Clifford Geertz (1973) has called "thick"; that is, it must be comprehensive and detailed, contain an adequate number of observations and widely sampled examples. Qualitative methods have very stringent criteria for determining data adequacy, and these should be followed. One of the most serious problems with the Wilsonian methods is that frequently analysts commence inquiry with a dictionary definition and use only one case study (often confabulated) to determine attributes, so that this approach fails to meet the first standard of data adequacy.

The second criterion is that, whatever methods are used, the researcher must demonstrate depth in the analysis. Intellectual rigor should be evident. The research must be logical, rigorous, and creative with a clearly developed and systematic presentation of the results. If this is absent (as with much of the research using Wilsonian methods), then such research will regularly fail to make any significant contribution.

Finally, the results should make a contribution to knowledge. The findings should make intuitive sense, in that they are recognizable, yet appear innovative. New concepts should provide new insights into phenomena and lead to

TABLE 4.7 Criteria for Evaluating Rigor of Concept Analysis Research

Criteria	Standard	
	Unacceptable	Acceptable
1. Extensiveness of the data base	Thin and scant Brief reports Recollected data Abbreviated case studies Confabulated examples	Rich and complete Loads of literature Full description Oodles of observations Widely sampled examples
2. Depth of analysis	Absent Trivial, insignificant Lacks depth	Intellectual rigor Logical Creative and original
3. Development of argument	Obsfucation Lacks reasoning	Logical Clarity
4. Validity	Lacks specificity to concept	Delineates inclusion/exclusion criteria
5. Level of abstractness	Context/situational bound	Encompasses all forms and situations of the concept
6. Contribution to knowledge	Findings are obvious Research does not contribute to the literature	Findings make intuitive sense Provides new insights and new perspectives into the phemonenon Empirical questions identifiable Facilitates inquiry

new areas of investigation by permitting the identification of empirical questions and facilitating inquiry. Recall, however, that all concepts are not immediately and equally mature; full maturity is achieved only over time, with continued use and refinement. New concepts should not be too quickly rated negatively simply because they fail to meet all of the above criteria, but should be considered in light of their potential contribution.

CONCLUSION

Concepts form the foundation of a discipline and the essence of the philosophical underpinnings that guide a profession. The strength of the theory that guides a discipline is dependent on the quality of its concepts and on the nature of the hypothesized relationships linking these concepts. Further, how the concepts are described, how the concepts are constructed, and how they are measured and manipulated in the clinical setting is dependent on the level of concept analysis in the discipline. Given the significance of concepts to a discipline, it is of serious concern that concepts used in nursing are relatively undeveloped and that its methods of concept analysis are still in their infancy. The movement from a pre-paradigmatic to a paradigmatic phase (Kuhn, 1970) in any research program will be dependent on concept formation that engages issues across the spectrum of concerns indicated by the epistemological, logical, pragmatic, and linguistic principles. But because of the lack of adequate and appropriate data, the lack of depth in analyses, the lack of reasoning, the lack of specificity, the absence of abstractness, and the minor contribution to knowledge derived from the use of Wilsonian-derived methods, we do not recommend the continued use of these methods for concept development.

REFERENCES

Allan, H. T. (1993). Feminism: A concept analysis. *Journal of Advanced Nursing, 18*, 1547-1553.

Applegate, M., & Morse, J. M. (1994). Personal privacy and interactional patterns in a nursing home. *Journal of Aging Studies, 8*(4), 413-434.

Arakelian, M. (1980). An assessment and nursing application of the concept of locus of control. *Advances in Nursing Science, 2*(1), 25-38.

Ashmore, R., & Ramsamy, S. (1993). The concept of the 'gaze' in mental health nursing. *Senior Nurse, 13*(1), 46-49.

Batey, M. Y. (1977). Conceptualization: Knowledge and logical grounding empirical research. *Nursing Research, 46*(5), 324-329.

Bolton, N. (1977). *Concept formation.* Oxford, England: Pergamon.

Boyd, C. (1985). Toward an understanding of mother-daughter identification using concept analysis. *Advances in Nursing Science, 7*(2), 78-85.

Campbell, L. (1987). Hopelessness. *Journal of Psychosocial Nursing, 25*(2), 18-29.

Caroline, H. (1993). Explorations of close friendship: A concept analysis. *Archives of Psychiatric Nursing, 7*(4), 236-243.

Chinn, P. L., & Jacobs, M. K. (1983). *Theory and nursing: A systematic approach.* St. Louis, MO: Mosby.

Chinn, P. L., & Jacobs, M. K. (1987). *Theory and nursing: A systematic approach.* (2nd ed.). St. Louis, MO: Mosby.

Chinn, P. L., & Kramer, M. K. (1991). *Theory and nursing: A systematic approach* (3rd ed.). St. Louis, MO: Mosby Year Book.

Cowles, K., & Rodgers, B. (1991). The concept of grief: A foundation for nursing research and practice. *Research in Nursing & Health, 14,* 119-127.

Crawford, G. (1982). The concept of pattern in nursing: Conceptual development and measurement. *Advances in Nursing Science, 4*(1), 1-6.

Estabrooks, C. A. (1989). Touch: A nursing strategy in the intensive care unit. *Heart & Lung, 18*(4), 392-401.

Estabrooks, C. A., & Morse, J. M. (1992). Toward a theory of touch: The touching process and acquiring a touching style. *Journal of Advanced Nursing, 17,* 448-456.

Ferrans, C. E., & Powers, M. J. (1992). Psychometric assessment of the quality of life index. *Research in Nursing & Health, 15,* 29-38.

Frost, M. H. (1992). Quality: A concept of importance to nursing. *Journal of Nursing Care Quality, 7*(1), 64-69.

Geertz, C. (1973). *The interpretation of cultures.* New York: Basic Books.

Geissler, E. (1984). Crisis: What it is and is not. *Advances in Nursing Science, 6*(1), 1-9.

Haase, J., Britt, T., Coward, D., Leidy, N. K., & Penn, P. (1992). Simultaneous concept analysis of spiritual perspective, hope, acceptance and self-transcendence. *Image: Journal of Nursing Scholarship, 24*(2), 141-147.

Hagerty, B., Lynch-Sauer, J., Patusky, K., Bouwsema, M., & Collier, P. (1992). Sense of belonging: A vital mental health concept. *Archives of Psychiatric Nursing, 6*(3), 172-177.

Hagerty, B., & Patusky, K. (1995). Developing a measure of sense of belonging. *Nursing Research, 44*(1), 9-13.

Hall, J. M., Stevens, P. E., & Meleis, A. I. (1994). Marginalization: A guiding concept for valuing diversity in nursing knowledge development. *Advances in Nursing Science, 16*(4), 23-41.

Hawks, J. H. (1991). Power: A concept analysis. *Journal of Advanced Nursing, 16,* 754-762.

Hawks, J. H. (1992). Empowerment in nursing education: Concept analysis and application to philosophy, learning and instruction. *Journal of Advanced Nursing, 17,* 609-618.

Hupcey, J., & Morse, J. M. (1995). *Social support: Assessing conceptual coherence.* Unpublished manuscript, The Pennsylvania State University, University Park, PA.

Jasper, M. (1994). Expert: A discussion of the implications of the concept as used in nursing. *Journal of Advanced Nursing, 20,* 769-776.

Jennings, B. M., & Staggers, N. (1994). A critical analysis of hardiness. *Nursing Research, 43*(5), 274-281.

Johnson, J. (1994). A dialectical examination of nursing art. *Advances in Nursing Science, 17*(1), 1-14.

Johnson, J., Ratner, P. A., Bottorff, J. L., & Hayduk, L. A. (1993). An exploration of Pender's Health Promotion Model using LISREL. *Nursing Research, 42*(3), 132-138.

Kolcaba, K. (1991). A taxonomic structure for the concept comfort. *Image: Journal of Nursing Scholarship, 23*(4), 237-240.
Kolcaba, K. (1992). The concept of comfort in an environmental framework. *Journal of Gerontological Nursing, 18*(6), 33-38.
Kolcaba, K., & Kolcaba, R. (1991). An analysis of the concept of comfort. *Journal of Advanced Nursing, 16*, 1301-1310.
Kuhn, T. (1970). *The structure of scientific revolutions* (2nd ed.). Chicago: University of Chicago Press.
La Monica, E. L. (1981). Construct validity of an empathy instrument. *Research in Nursing and Health, 4*, 389-400.
Lindgren, C., Burke, M., Hainsworth, M., & Eakes, G. (1992). Chronic sorrow: A lifespan concept. *Scholarly Inquiry for Nursing Practice, 6*(1), 27-40.
Lützén, K., & Nordin, C. (1993). Benevolence, a central moral concept derived from a grounded theory study of nursing decision making in psychiatric settings. *Journal of Advanced Nursing, 18*, 1106-1111.
Madden, B. (1990). The hybrid model for concept development: Its value for the study of therapeutic alliance. *Advances in Nursing Science, 12*(3), 75-87.
Mahon, N. E., & Yarcheski, A. (1988). Loneliness in early adolescents: An empirical test of alternate explanations. *Nursing Research, 37*(6), 330-335.
Mairis, E. (1994). Concept clarification in professional practice—dignity. *Journal of Advanced Nursing, 19*, 947-953.
Matteson, P., & Hawkins, J. (1990). Concept analysis of decision making. *Nursing Forum, 25*(2), 4-10.
Meeberg, G. (1993). Quality of life: A concept analysis. *Journal of Advanced Nursing, 18*, 32-38.
Meize-Grochowski, R. (1984). An analysis of the concept of trust. *Journal of Advanced Nursing, 9*, 563-572.
Mercer, R. T., & Ferketich, S. L. (1994). Predictors of maternal role competence by risk status. *Nursing Research, 42*(1), 38-43.
Miller, J. F., & Powers, M. J. (1988). Development of an instrument to measure hope. *Nursing Research, 37*(1), 6-10.
Mishel, M. H. (1981). The measurement of uncertainty in illness. *Nursing Research, 30*(5), 258-263.
Mishel, M. H. (1983). Parents' perceptions of uncertainty concerning their hospitalized child. *Nursing Research, 32*(6), 324-330.
Mishel, M. H. (1984). Perceived uncertainty and stress in illness. *Research in Nursing and Health, 7*, 163-171.
Mishel, M. H., & Braden, C. J. (1988). Finding meaning: Antecedents of uncertainty in illness. *Nursing Research, 37*(2), 98-103, 127.
Mishel, M. H., Padilla, G., Grant, M., & Sorenson, D. S. (1991). Uncertainty in illness theory: A replication of the mediating effects of mastery and coping. *Nursing Research, 40*(4), 236-240.
Morse, J. M. (1987). The meaning of health in an inner city community. *Nursing Papers, 19*(2), 27-41.
Morse, J. M. (1994). Compathy. Unpublished manuscript, The Pennsylvania State University, University Park, PA.
Morse, J. M. (1995). Exploring the theoretical basis of nursing using advanced techniques of concept analysis. *Advances in Nursing Science, 17*(3), 31-46.
Morse, J. M. (in review). Nursing scholarship: Sense and sensibility. *Nursing Inquiry.*
Morse, J. M., Anderson, G., Bottorff, J., Yonge, O., O'Brien, B., Solberg, S., & McIlveen, K. H. (1992). Exploring empathy: A conceptual fit for nursing practice? *Image: Journal of Nursing Scholarship, 24*(4), 273-280.

Morse, J. M., Bottorff, J., Anderson, G., O'Brien, B., & Solberg, S. (1992). Beyond empathy: Expanding expressions of caring. *Journal of Advanced Nursing, 17,* 809-821.

Morse, J. M., Bottorff, J., Neander, W., & Solberg, S. (1991). Comparative analysis of the conceptualizations and theories of caring. *Image: Journal of Nursing Scholarship, 23*(2), 119-126.

Morse, J. M., & Carter, B. (1996). The essence of enduring and the expression of suffering: The reformulation of self. *Scholarly Inquiry for Nursing Practice, 10*(1), 43-60.

Morse, J. M., & Doberneck, B. M. (in press). Delineating the concept of hope. *Image: Journal of Nursing Scholarship.*

Morse, J. M., Miles, M., Clark, D., & Doberneck, B. (1994). "Sensing" patient needs: Exploring concepts of nursing insight and receptivity used in nursing assessment. *Scholarly Inquiry for Nursing Practice, 8*(3), 233-260.

Morse, J. M., Mitcham, C., Hupcey, J. E., & Tasón, M. C. (1996). Criteria for concept evaluation. *Journal of Advanced Nursing, 24*(2), 385-390.

Morse, J. M., Solberg, S., Neander, W., Bottorff, J., & Johnson, J. (1990). Concepts of caring and caring as a concept. *Advances in Nursing Science, 13*(1), 1-14.

Nemcek, M. A. (1987). Self nurturing: A concept analysis. *American Association of Occupational Health Nurses Journal, 35*(8), 349-352.

Norbeck, J. S., Lindsey, A. M., & Carrieri, V. L. (1981). The development of an instrument to measure social support. *Nursing Research, 30*(5), 264-269.

Norbeck, J. S., Lindsey, A. M., & Carrieri, V. L. (1983). Further development of the Norbeck social support questionnaire: Normative data and validity testing. *Nursing Research, 32*(1), 4-9.

Owen, D. (1989). Nurses' perspectives on the meaning of hope in patients with cancer: A qualitative study. *Oncology Nurses Forum, 16*(1), 75-79.

Panzarine, S. (1985). Coping: Conceptual and methodological issues. *Advances in Nursing Science, 7*(4), 49-57.

Payne, L. (1983). Health: A basic concept in nursing theory. *Journal of Advanced Nursing, 8,* 393-395.

Phillips, M. (1991). Chronic sorrow in mothers of chronically ill and disabled children. *Issues in Comprehensive Pediatric Nursing, 14,* 111-120.

Quinless, F. W., McDermott, & Nelson, M. A. (1988). Development of a measure of learned helplessness. *Nursing Research, 37*(1), 11-15.

Ratner, P. A., Bottorff, J. L., Johnson, J. L., & Hayduk, L. A. (in press). Using multiple indicators to test the dimensionality of concepts. *Research in Nursing and Health.*

Rawnsley, M. M. (1980). The concept of privacy. *Advances in Nursing Science, 2*(2), 25-31.

Reed, P., & Leonard, V. (1989). An analysis of the concept of self-neglect. *Advances in Nursing Science, 12*(1), 39-53.

Rew, L. (1986). Intuition: Concept analysis of a group phenomenon. *Advances in Nursing Science, 8*(2), 21-28.

Roberts, K., & Fitzgerald, L. (1991). Serenity: Caring with perspective. *Scholarly Inquiry for Nursing Practice, 5*(2), 127-146.

Rodgers, B. (1989). Exploring health policy as a concept. *Western Journal of Nursing Research, 11*(6), 694-702.

Rodgers, B. L. (1993). Concept analysis: An evolutionary view. In B. L. Rodgers & K. A. Knafl (Eds.), *Concept development in nursing* (pp. 73-92). Philadelphia: Saunders.

Rodgers, B., & Cowles, K. (1991). The concept of grief: An analysis of classical and contemporary thought. *Death Studies, 15,* 443-458.

Sarkis, J., & Skoner, M. (1987). An analysis of the concept of holism in nursing literature. *Holistic Nursing Practice, 2*(1), 61-69.

Schwartz-Barcott, D., & Kim, H. S. (1986). A hybrid model for concept development. In P. L. Chinn (Ed.), *Nursing research methodology: Issues and implementations* (pp. 91- 101). Rockville, MD: Aspen.

Schwartz-Barcott, D., & Kim, H. S. (1993). An expansion and elaboration of the hybrid model of concept development. In B. L. Rodgers & K. A. Knafl (Eds.), *Concept development in nursing* (pp. 107-133). Philadelphia: Saunders.

Simmons, S. (1989). Health: A concept analysis. *International Journal of Nursing Studies, 26*(2), 155-161.

Stephenson, C. (1991). The concept of hope revisited for nursing. *Journal of Advanced Nursing, 16*, 1456-1461.

Teasdale, K. (1989). The concept of reassurance in nursing. *Journal of Advanced Nursing, 14*, 444-450.

Teel, C. (1991). Chronic sorrow: Analysis of the concept. *Journal of Advanced Nursing, 16*, 1311-1319.

Timmerman, G. (1991). A concept analysis of intimacy. *Issues in Mental Health Nursing, 12*, 19-30.

Trandel-Korenchuk, D. (1986). Concept development in nursing research. *Nursing Administration Quarterly, 11*(1), 1-9.

Tuck, I., & Keels, M. (1992). Milieu therapy: A review of development of this concept and its implications for psychiatric nursing. *Issues in Mental Health Nursing, 13*, 51-58.

van Manen, M. (1991). *The tact of teaching: The meaning of pedagogical thoughtfulness.* Albany, NY: State University of New York Press

Verhulst, G., & Schwartz-Barcott, D. (1993). A concept analysis of withdrawal: Application of the hybrid model of concept development. In B. Rodgers & K. Knafl (Eds.), *Concept development in nursing* (pp. 135-157). Philadelphia: W. B. Saunders.

Walker, L. O., & Avant, K. C. (1983). *Strategies for theory construction in nursing.* Norwalk, CT: Appleton-Century-Crofts.

Walker, L. O., & Avant, K. C. (1988). *Strategies for theory construction in nursing* (2nd ed.). Norwalk, CT: Appleton-Century-Crofts.

Walker, L. O., & Avant, K. C. (1995). *Strategies for theory construction in nursing* (3rd ed.). Norwalk, CT: Appleton-Century-Crofts.

Wallace, W. A. (1983). Basic concepts: Natural and scientific. In *From a realist point of view* (pp. 45-69). Lanham, MD: University Press of America.

Waltz, C. F., Strickland, O. L., & Lenz, E. R. (1991). *Measurement in nursing research* (2nd ed.). Philadelphia: F. A. Davis.

Warren, B. J. (1993). Explaining social isolation through concept analysis. *Archives of Psychiatric Nursing, 7*(5), 270-276.

Wartofsky, M. W. (1968). *Conceptual foundations of scientific thought: An introduction to the philosophy of science.* New York: Macmillan.

Watson, S. (1991). An analysis of the concept of experience. *Journal of Advanced Nursing, 16*, 1117-1121.

Westra, B., & Rodgers, B. (1991). The concept of integration: A foundation for evaluating outcomes of nursing care. *Journal of Professional Nursing, 7*(5), 277-282.

Wilson, J. (1969). *Thinking with concepts.* Cambridge, England: Cambridge University Press. (Original work published in 1963)

Yoder, L. (1990). Mentoring: A concept analysis. *Nursing Administration Quarterly, 15*(1), 9-19.

Younger, J. (1991). A theory of mastery. *Advances in Nursing Science, 14*(1), 76-89.

5

Postpartum Fatigue: Clarifying a Concept

Renee Milligan, PhD, RN
Elizabeth R. Lenz, Ph.D, RN, FAAN
Peggy L. Parks, PhD
Linda C. Pugh, PhD, RNC
Harriet Kitzman, PhD, RN

Postpartum fatigue is a common occurrence that is often discussed in casual conversation by laypersons and health professionals. Like many concepts that are central to nursing, it is part of the common parlance, and its meaning is assumed to be clear and mutually understood by those using the term. As nurses work to develop and refine the science, however, it is essential to scrutinize such concepts carefully for consistency and completeness of meaning in various clinical populations and contexts, that is, consistency and completeness of definitions and dimensions, clarity of boundaries and indicators, and the existence of clear clinical exemplars.

To date, concept analyses by nurses have tended to focus on literary approaches, with most using adaptations of the procedure recommended by Wilson (1963) (see Hupcey, Morse, Lenz, & Tasón, in chapter 1). With the exception of the nursing measurement literature and Morse's (e.g., Morse, 1995; Morse & Carter, 1996; Morse, Solberg, Neander, Bottorff, & Johnson, 1990; Morse & Doberneck, 1996) use of qualitative research for analyzing selected psychosocial concepts, there has been surprisingly little empirically based concept analysis and development work reported.

This chapter describes a multifaceted approach to concept clarification which was applied over a decade by the first author and her collaborators. The

Acknowledgment. The authors wish to acknowledge the assistance of Sister Mary Jean Flaherty, Dean, School of Nursing, The Catholic University of America, as the content analysis of the qualitative data progressed.

target concept was postpartum fatigue; this was later expanded to the more encompassing concept, childbearing fatigue. The process began with a literary analysis of the concept, but then went beyond the literature to a series of related studies, both qualitative and quantitative. The studies have addressed such issues as identifying commonly experienced indicators or referents and differentiation from related concepts. The approach described here evolved as empirical findings about fatigue generated some answers and many new questions.

BEGINNING STAGES: ANALYSIS OF EXISTING LITERATURE

The first author's interest in the concept of postpartum fatigue began in 1985 and was based on years of clinical experience with new mothers. Of particular interest was the question of whether the common phenomenon of "baby blues" is, in fact, maternal fatigue. Guidance for beginning the initial analysis of the concept was provided by Norris's (1982) book, *Concept Clarification*. Norris organized diverse phenomena under the rubric of "basic physiological protection mechanisms" (p. 385), one of which was fatigue.

The first step was to analyze and evaluate the existing literature. Evaluation of available nursing literature revealed insufficient information to permit a deductive approach, such as theory testing. A thorough literature search failed to identify studies specifically about postpartum fatigue; however, in the nonempirical maternity nursing literature it was identified as a concern to new mothers. The literature review revealed limitations on the quality of measurement of fatigue. Investigators had identified the existence of postpartum fatigue largely by responses to lists of concerns (e.g., Fawcett & York, 1986; Harrison & Hicks, 1983; Hiser, 1987). Qualitative descriptions of experience were also used to identify fatigue (e.g., Chapman, Macey, Keegan, Borum, & Bennett, 1985; Fawcett, 1981; Mercer, 1986; Merilo, 1988).

Given the immature development of the concept, the literary analysis was broadened to include fatigue (not necessarily postpartum) in the disciplines of ergonomics, medicine, industry and psychology. Detailed results of this analysis have been published elsewhere (Milligan & Pugh, 1994). Some key questions about the concept of fatigue were identified as needing clarification, and these questions served as the bases for subsequent empirical study. The questions are listed below, and aspects of the 1985 "state of the science" that gave rise to them are briefly described.

1. Does the concept fatigue differ from the concepts of tiredness or weariness? Do new mothers describe fatigue to be different from normal tiredness?

According to Bartley (1976) and Broadbent (1979), the term fatigue evolved as a more formal way of conveying tiredness or weariness. Initially, therefore, it was used synonymously with these terms. Later, fatigue and normal tiredness began to be differentiated from one another, with fatigue designating a phenomenon that is more severe and longer lasting. For example, Morris (1982) noted that fatigue (versus tiredness) is present when usual recovery modes, such as a night's sleep, are not effective in restoring vigor. Whether new mothers describe their feelings as more severe than normal tiredness needed to be ascertained.

2. What are the defining characteristics of fatigue and of postpartum fatigue? Is fatigue most meaningfully portrayed as a general state or as a complex of discrete feelings?

The term fatigue was used initially to encompass a wide range of feelings and behaviors, including feeling all tired out, weary, unable to sustain interest and effort, and lazy; as well as difficulty with performing tasks, decreased work productivity, and diminished capacity for living (Burkhardt, 1956). Later, a more sophisticated notion evolved, with feelings and behaviors beginning to be differentiated. For example, Yoshitake (1971), who had done extensive work on the definition and measurement of fatigue of industrial workers in Japan, conceptualized fatigue as a complex of unpleasant feelings such as aversion to work, wish for rest, impatience, drowsiness and dullness, difficulty in concentrating, projection of physical impairment, and incongruous physical, mental and sensory-neurological feelings. He identified three patterns or clusters of these symptoms as drowsiness and dullness, difficulty of concentration, and projection of physical impairment (Yoshitake, 1978). He claimed that the symptoms of fatigue are similar to, but not the same as, a general feeling of fatigue. The scale that he developed to measure fatigue in Japanese industrial workers was a checklist of specific symptoms or indicators.

3. Can fatigue/postpartum fatigue and depression be differentiated theoretically and empirically?

An important issue for concept clarification that surfaced in the literature review was the relationship and potential conceptual overlap between fatigue and depression. Fatigue was most often identified to be a symptom of depression or anxiety, and was included on diagnostic assessment tools as an indicator of these conditions (e.g., Beck, Ward, Mendelson, Mack, & Erbaugh, 1961; Radloff, 1977). Conversely, Montgomery (1983) and Rhoten (1982) found negative psychologic states, such as depression and/or somatic anxiety, to be prevalent in persons who are fatigued. Hargreaves (1977) defined the "fatigue syndrome" as indistinguishable from an anxiety state with depressive features. In some literature, fatigue and depression were depicted as related but distinctive concepts (e.g., Robson, 1982). The extent to which fatigue and depressive symptomology are distinct phenomena in new mothers needed to be clarified.

CLARIFYING QUALITIES AND CORRELATES OF POSTPARTUM FATIGUE

In order to begin to answer the above questions regarding the nature of postpartum fatigue two studies—one qualitative the other quantitative—were undertaken simultaneously. The study sample for the quantitative analysis was a subsample ($n = 285$)[1] from a larger sample of new mothers participating in a longitudinal (18-month) study by Parks and Lenz[2] of predictors of maternal behavior and infant development. The study sample for the qualitative study was a convenience subsample ($n = 55$) of the mothers who participated in the quantitative study. These primiparous and multiparous mothers were White, ranged in age from 18 to 37 and from low to high socioeconomic status (SES). The majority had had vaginal deliveries, were married, and were bottle feeding their infants.

Mothers' Qualitative Descriptions

The qualitative study (see Milligan, 1989) took place when the 55 subjects were 3 months postpartum. The purpose of the study was to clarify the nature of postpartum fatigue from the mother's perspective. During home interviews mothers were first asked to rate their level of tiredness on a visual analog scale. Using this level as a reference point, they were then asked to describe their tiredness or fatigue in detail, and to clarify how it differed from the "blues. " The terms tiredness and fatigue were intentionally used together by the investigator, in order to allow mothers either to use them synonymously or to differentiate them. Fifty-two responses were transcribed, coded, and analyzed using Patton's (1980) method for analysis of text. Four major themes emerged: two represented characteristics and two represented causes of postpartal fatigue. The results of the qualitative study were particularly helpful in addressing the question about the distinctions between postpartum fatigue and depression.

The themes, manifestations and normalcy, describe mothers' perceptions of being fatigued. The characteristics were both physical and psychological, and many were quite specific, e.g., "I want to sit down. " Psychologically oriented descriptions were typically related to the differences or similarities between fatigue and depression. For example, "Blues is sadness, not tiredness," or "When you're depressed, you cannot cope; when you're tired, you still do things. " More rarely, but also more important, mothers related high fatigue to depression, e.g., "When you get overly tired, you get depressed. " It seemed easy for mothers to discern the difference between low or moderate levels of fatigue and "blues"; however, if fatigue was high, the feeling was more similar to depression.

Normalcy represented the mothers' perceptions that the fatigue they were experiencing was a transitory state; that is, if they returned to normal routines, their fatigue would decrease or disappear. Mothers perceived their fatigue as a temporary condition that would go away if they could only get organized, get on a schedule, or get back to their usual sleep patterns. For example, "I know when we settle down, the fatigue's going to go away." These remarks suggest that postpartum fatigue differs from the tiredness that had been experienced in other circumstances, and is a temporary state from which mothers will eventually emerge.

The two themes representing perceived causes of postpartum fatigue were family management and pile-up. Aspects of the new mothers' lives that were intrinsic to caring for their families were perceived to cause fatigue. Mothers addressed such factors as the baby's sleep–wake cycle, housework, lack of partner support, responsibility to other children and infant feeding. Often the idea that mothers should expect to be tired was reflected in the text. For example, "Being a mother with two kids, you know, sometimes I'm up with him, with his feedings and things. And then I'm up at 7:00, 8:00 in the morning when she gets up. You know, that's about all; it's just typical tiredness." This mother did not differentiate normal tiredness from fatigue; however, many mothers did convey the idea that the postpartal fatigue they were experiencing was more severe and prolonged than tiredness they had experienced prior to the pregnancy.

The theme pile-up, although it included the mothers' caregiving roles, also included roles external to the family and reflected the idea that the demands of multiple roles accumulate. Mothers described being overextended, for example, "overworked," "overwhelmed by all the different things I was trying to do,"and facing "more than I can ever get done." Both family management and pile-up themes suggest the importance of the social context in influencing levels of fatigue.

Indicators and Predictors of Postpartal Fatigue: Quantitative Analyses

The first of several quantitative studies to discern the nature of postpartum fatigue was carried out simultaneously with the qualitative study using a subsample of the Parks and Lenz data set comprised of 259 lower and middle SES mothers (see Milligan, 1989; Milligan, Parks, & Lenz, 1990). A modification of Yoshitake's (1971) Fatigue Symptoms Checklist (named the Modified Fatigue Symptoms Checklist—MFSC) was administered within 24 hours following delivery and at 6 weeks and 3 months postpartum. The scale lists 30 indicators of fatigue, each of which respondents self-report as present or absent at the time the scale is completed. At 3 months the mothers also rated their tiredness on a visual analog scale; at all time periods their depressive symptoms were measured using the Center for Epidemiologic Studies Depression Scale (CES-D) (Radloff, 1977).

Mothers reported an average of 7.05 (SD = 4.62) on the MFSC shortly following delivery, 7.58 (SD = 5.20) at 6 weeks and 5.80 (SD = 4.56) at 3 months postpartum, with a range from 0 to 28. A major emphasis of the analysis was to discern predictors of postpartum fatigue at each of the three time periods. With depressive symptomology controlled in a hierarchical stepwise multiple regression, it was found that type of delivery predicted fatigue immediately postpartum, with higher fatigue being associated with surgical (versus vaginal) delivery. Infant difficulty (score on the "difficulty" subscale of the Bates Infant Characteristics Questionnaire (Bates, Freeland, & Lounsbury, 1979) and type of infant feeding (breast versus bottle) were predictors of fatigue at 6 weeks postpartum. Infant difficulty continued to predict fatigue at 3 months postpartum, as did SES, with higher fatigue associated with higher status. An interesting pattern that emerged from the analysis was that physical factors (type of delivery and infant feeding) played a more influential role in fatigue at early stages of the postpartal period, and social environmental factors (infant difficulty and socioeconomic status) became more important over time.

The total MFSC score correlated with the visual analog scale for tiredness ($r = .595$, $p < .001$), suggesting that there is a moderately high degree of correspondence—but not a complete overlap—between global ratings of tiredness and the occurrence of specific fatigue symptoms. It was unclear from this analysis whether the global rating or the summated rating of separate symptoms more appropriately represented the concept of postpartum fatigue, and, if the latter, which indicators should be considered core.

Dimensions of Fatigue: Factor Analysis

In order to pursue the above questions regarding the indicators of fatigue, another secondary analysis of the data set from the Parks and Lenz study was carried out using factor analysis. The idea that fatigue can be represented by a single global rating suggests that it is essentially unidimensional. The alternative conceptualization is that it has several dimensions that would be expected to emerge as independent factors. Factor analyses of the MFSC data for 285 mothers at the immediate postpartum period and at 6 weeks and 3 months after delivery revealed a pattern of two clusters of indicators that were consistent across all three time periods. These were labeled mental fatigue and physical fatigue. The indicators of mental fatigue were "my head feels heavy," "my brain feels hot or muddled," "it's difficult to think," "I get weary talking," "I can't concentrate," and "I am apt to forget things." The indicators of physical fatigue are "my body feels tired," "my legs feel tired," "I am drowsy," and "I want to lie down" (Milligan, Parks, Lenz, & Kitzman, in review). The extraction of two consistent factors suggests that it may be more meaningful to portray fatigue as clusters of indicators than as a global, unidimensional construct.

Correlates of Physical and Mental Fatigue

Given the finding that physical and mental fatigue represent two independent dimensions that could be considered different types of fatigue, additional clarification was needed about whether the two types are distinct. Milligan and Kitzman

(1992) studied fatigue in 74 low-income, urban dwelling, predominantly African American mothers across the three trimesters of pregnancy and at 6 months postpartum. Lending support to the validity of the distinction, they found that anxiety, depression, and conflict with those in mothers' support networks were more strongly correlated with mental than with physical fatigue. They also found that activities regarding child care, such as expectations of support for child care and perceived efficacy in performing child-care functions, were negatively correlated with physical fatigue but were not correlated with mental fatigue. This finding is consistent with the labor-intensive nature of child care, which is generally more demanding physically than mentally. The findings from this study also began to provide limited evidence for the generalizability of the earlier findings regarding an exclusively White sample to mothers of other racial groups.

DIFFERENTIATING FATIGUE AND DEPRESSION

One of the most compelling questions regarding the concept of fatigue is the nature of its overlap with depression, and much of the work of concept clarification has focused on this issue. Although postpartum fatigue is sometimes identified as a symptom of depression, the a priori assumption was made that the two concepts are potentially distinguishable. To determine the extent to which this assumption is valid in postpartum mothers, two questions were addressed in a secondary analysis of the data from the 285 mothers used in the Parks and Lenz data set (Milligan, Parks, & Lenz, 1993). The first question was whether fatigue and depression change differently over the first 3 months of the postpartum period. Using repeated measures analyses of covariance, with first one concept then the other dependent and the other a covariate, followed by post hoc Tukey tests, it was found that the patterns of change, in fact, differed. The level of fatigue (with depression controlled) changed significantly across the three measurement periods. Levels of fatigue were significantly higher immediately after delivery and at 6 weeks postpartum (when they were highest) than at 3 months postpartum. Depression (with fatigue controlled),however, did not change significantly over time. The dissimilar patterns of change over time supported the idea that each of the concepts is distinct.

The second question related to the differential prediction of fatigue and depression: do different variables predict fatigue than predict depression? At each measurement period, relevant demographic, clinical, and situational characteristics (e.g., maternal age, socioeconomic status, parity, type of delivery, type of feeding, and infant difficulty) were identified as possible predictors. Separate hierarchial multiple regression analyses were conducted at each time period and for each of the two concepts as criterion variables. With fatigue dependent, two different analyses were conducted at each time period. First, a stepwise multiple regression was carried out with the possible predictor variables, but without depression included. A second analysis was then carried out in which depression was statistically controlled by entering it on the first step, then entering the other predictors in a stepwise fashion. Parallel analyses were carried out with depression dependent.

Results from this study, which are more extensive than discussed here, revealed different predictors for depression and fatigue, supporting the conclusion that the two concepts are distinct. For instance, at the immediate postpartum period, type of delivery predicted fatigue with depression controlled; however, there were no significant predictors of depression. At 6 weeks and 3 months, infant difficulty was a predictor of fatigue with depression controlled, but was not a predictor of depression. At 6 weeks, breast feeding was associated with higher levels of fatigue (with depression controlled), but bottle feeding was associated with higher levels of depression (with fatigue controlled).

The analysis also revealed some interesting comparisons between analyses with and without the respective concept controlled. At the immediate postpartum period, when depression was dependent without controlling fatigue, the significant predictors were maternal age and type of delivery. When fatigue was controlled, thus removing the variance in depression attributable to it, no significant predictors remained. This finding suggests two explanations that need to be examined in future research: (1) either fatigue accounts for so much of the variance in depression that, once held constant, there is little variance left to be explained or predicted by other variables; or (2) fatigue mediates the relationships between the predictors and depression, i. e., the predictors of depression work by influencing the level of fatigue which, in turn, influences depression.

MODEL DEVELOPMENT

Following the initial literary, qualitative and quantitative analyses, Milligan (1989) developed a working definition and model of postpartum fatigue. Her early definition of fatigue was similar to that developed by Yoshitake (1971, 1978): "a subjective state of feeling tired. It can range in intensity on a continuum from feeling slightly tired to feeling completely exhausted... Fatigue is manifest in a variety of nonspecific subjectively perceived symptoms of drowsiness and dullness, difficulty in concentration, and physical impairment. These symptoms are similar to, but not the same as, an overall feeling of tiredness" (p. 11).

The model was a Venn diagram in which postpartum fatigue is depicted by a large circle that overlaps a second circle representing maternal depressive symptomology. The nonoverlapping portion of the postpartum fatigue circle represents that portion of the concept's meaning that is distinct from depressive symptoms. Likewise, the nonoverlapping portion of the circle representing depressive symptomology is the distinct core of that concept. Consistent with qualitative interview data and the findings from the MFSC, the fatigue circle is labeled to include both physical and psychological manifestations. Continued clarification of the concept of postpartum fatigue has substantiated that the essential elements of this very preliminary model remain valid, but need to be more fully elaborated. Empirical findings indicated a need to change the definition. For example, it was apparent that tiredness should not be considered analogous to fatigue, and that reference to the three clusters of symptoms should be omitted.

Model development activities continued in collaboration with Pugh (1990) whose study of 100 women during labor and the immediate postpartum period revealed that fatigue was cumulative and that women admitted to labor with high levels of fatigue, tended to have higher fatigue as labor progressed. Pugh and Milligan (1993) developed a model of childbearing fatigue that encompasses pregnancy and labor, as well as the postpartum period. The model builds upon and extends Milligan's earlier work by addressing "causes" and consequences of fatigue. It portrays that at each period of childbearing a variety of physiological, psychological and situational factors impact fatigue which, in turn, influences performance. The model highlights the importance of distinguishing between the experience of fatigue and its effect on the mother's performance, including the work of labor and the many aspects of the maternal role.

In the Pugh and Milligan (1993) model, the North American Nursing Diagnosis Association's (NANDA) definition of fatigue was used as the conceptual definition. Fatigue was defined as "an overwhelming sustained sense of exhaustion and decreased capacity for physical and mental work. " Consistent with Milligan's earlier research, this definition depicts fatigue as an unpleasant sensation that, if allowed to continue, leads to exhaustion. It, thus, excludes the more positive feelings that can occur when one is tired, yet invigorated, e.g., the good feeling after exercise, or the satisfied feeling of a job well done. Also consistent with empirical findings is the inclusion of reference to physical and mental manifestations of fatigue. However, it is unclear whether in the NANDA definition, " capacity for physical and mental work" refers to a behavioral manifestation or a behavioral consequence of fatigue. If the latter, then the definition seems inconsistent with the Pugh and Milligan model's separation of feelings/sensations (the experience of fatigue) and behavior (performance). Further study and clarification are needed, including differentiating behavioral manifestations and behavioral outcomes of fatigue.

CONCLUSION

This chapter exemplifies an approach to concept development and clarification that goes beyond the Wilsonian method by employing a combination of literary and empirical analyses. Questions raised by the initial review of the literature about postpartum fatigue were used as the basis for empirical research, which, in turn, raised more questions about the nature of the concept. After a decade of work, the concept of postpartum fatigue has not been definitively "mapped" (see Waltz, Strickland, & Lenz, 1991), but some strides have been made. For example:

1. It seems clear that while the terms fatigue (or postpartum/childbearing fatigue) and tiredness are used synonymously by lay persons, the two concepts are not identical and should be differentiated in nursing's scientific lexicon. The former is more severe and prolonged, is a negative feeling, and is not as easily relieved.

2. Postpartum fatigue is more effectively conceptualized as a multidimensional concept with physical/physiological and mental/psychological aspects than as a global concept. Physical and mental fatigue during pregnancy and the postpartum are predicted by different variables; therefore, differentiating the two types may help in designing more specific and effective interventions. Although there is a moderately high relationship between global, single-item ratings of fatigue and summed ratings based on specific indicators, it is more meaningful to use multiple-item measures that address both physical and mental/psychological manifestations.

3. Postpartum fatigue and depression (and/or the less severe "baby blues") are distinct concepts that overlap somewhat in meaning and in measurable indicators. Evidence that they are distinct was provided by their dissimilar patterns of change over the postpartum, the different patterns of prediction, and the clear ability of postpartum women to differentiate them. Evidence for overlap was provided by some mothers who used the terms interchangeably and by the moderately high correlation between measures of the two concepts, possibly partially an artifact of the instruments used. Continued conceptual and empirical clarification is needed. Particular attention needs to be paid to selecting or developing measurement tools that do not overlap and to empirically test the role of fatigue as a mediator between mothers' physical, emotional, and situational variables and level of depressive symptomology.

As concept clarification activities continue, it will be essential to assure that empirical and conceptual/theoretical developments proceed and are integrated with one another and with practice. Theoretical models of the concept must be revised continually to incorporate empirical findings. Present models do not adequately reflect the nature and complexity of postpartum fatigue, and development needs to continue. The Pugh and Milligan (1993) model acknowledges the importance of antecedents and consequences, but does not adequately represent the complexity of the fatigue experience itself. The nature of fatigue as multidimensional and as overlapping with related variables is more effectively portrayed by the earlier Milligan (1989) model. The two might be combined and additional studies conducted that will be useful in more fully elaborating the concept's antecedent factors and its boundaries and relationships with other concepts, such as anxiety. It will be important to seek additional clarification and consistency about whether definitions of postpartum/childbearing fatigue should include behaviors as essential characteristics or be limited to sensations.

Because nursing is a scientific discipline, its key concepts need to be clearly, carefully and thoroughly delineated. Reliance on common parlance simply is not sufficient. Yet, because nursing is a practice discipline, its science also needs to be reality based. It is not sufficient to rely on hypothetical cases and literary analysis. The approach to concept development and clarification exemplified here is promising, because it shifts between the theoretical and empirical, the abstract and the real, to move the science forward in a meaningful and useful way.

NOTES

[1] Due to the small number of high SES subjects, some analyses carried out with this data set were conducted with only those 259 mothers who were middle and lower SES.
[2] Parks, P. L., Principal Investigator, and Lenz, E. R., Co-Principal Investigator. "Predictors of Maternal Behavior and Child Development. " Grant #R01NR01239, National Center for Nursing Research, 9/1/86 - 8/31/90.

REFERENCES

Bartley, S. H. (1976). What do we call fatigue? In E. Simonson & P. C. Weiser, *Psychological aspects and physiological correlates of work and fatigue* (pp. 409-414). Springfield, IL: Charles C. Thomas.

Bates, J., Freeland, C., & Lounsbury, M. (1979). Measurement of infant difficulties. *Child Development, 50,* 794-803.

Beck, A. T., Ward, C. H., Mendelson, M., Mock, J., & Erbaugh, J. (1961). An inventory for measuring depression. *Archives of General Psychiatry, 4,* 561-565.

Broadbent, D. E. (1979). Is a fatigue test now possible? *Ergonomics, 22,* 1277-1290.

Burkhardt, E. A. (1956, January 1). Fatigue—diagnosis and treatment. *New York State Journal of Medicine, 56*(1), 62-67.

Chapman, J. J., Macey, M. J., Keegan, M., Borum, P., & Bennett, S. (1985). Concerns of breast-feeding mothers from birth to 4 months. *Nursing Research, 34,* 374-377.

Fawcett, J. (1981). Needs of cesarean birth parents. *JOGNN: Journal of Obstetrics, Gynecologic, and Neonatal Nursing, 10*(5), 372-376.

Fawcett, J., & York, R. (1986). Spouses' physical and psychological symptoms during pregnancy and the postpartum. *Nursing Research, 35,* 144-146.

Hargreaves, M. (1977). The fatigue syndrome. *Practitioner, 218,* 841-843.

Harrison, M. J., & Hicks, S. A. (1983). Postpartum concerns of mothers and their sources of help. *Canadian Journal of Public Health, 74,* 325-327.

Hiser, P. L. (1987). Concerns of multiparas during the second postpartum week. *Journal of Gynecologic and Neonatal Nursing, 16,* 195-203.

Hupcey, J., Morse, J. M., Lenz, E. R., & Tasón, M. C. (1996). Wilsonian methods of concept analysis: A critique. *Scholarly Inquiry for Nursing Practice, 19*(3), 185-210.

Hart, L. K., & Freel, M. I. (1982). Fatigue. In C. Norris (Ed.), *Concept clarification in nursing* (pp. 251-262). Rockville, MD: Aspen.

Mercer, R. T. (1986). *First-time motherhood: Experiences from teens to forties.* New York: Springer Publishing Company.

Merilo, K. F. (1988). Is it better the second time around? *MCN: American Journal of Maternal Child Nursing, 13,* 200-204.

Mills, M., Arnold, B., & Wood, C. M. (1983). Core-12: A controlled study of 12-hour scheduling. *Nursing Research, 32,* 356-361.

Milligan, R. (1989). Maternal fatigue during the first three months of the postpartum period. *Dissertation Abstracts International, 50,* 07-B.

Milligan, R. (1990, May). Why am I so tired? A study of new mothers. Poster presented at The Ohio State University College of Nursing, The Ohio State University Hospitals Division of Nursing, and Columbus Children's Hospital, "Integrating Nursing Research and Practice, Visions for the Future," Columbus, OH.

Milligan, R., & Kitzman, H. (1992, March). *Fatigue during pregnancy.* Presentation at Nursing Research Across the Life Span: Methods, Issues and Interventions, sponsored by the Johns Hopkins University and University of Maryland at Baltimore, Baltimore, MD.

Milligan, R., Parks, P., & Lenz, E. (1990). An analysis of postpartum fatigue over the first three months of the postpartum period. In J.F. Wang, P.S. Simoni, & C.L. Nath (Eds.), *Proceedings of the West Virginia nurses' association 1990 research symposium.*

Milligan, R. A., Parks, P., & Lenz, E. (1993, November). *Distinguishing between postpartum depression and postpartum fatigue.* Paper presented at the American Nurses Association Council of Nurse Researchers Scientific Sessions. Washington, DC.

Milligan, R., Parks, P., Lenz, E., & Kitzman, H. (in review). Measuring women's fatigue during the postpartum period.

Milligan, R., & Pugh, L. (1994). Fatigue during the childbearing period. *Annual Review of Nursing Research, 12,* 33-49.

Montgomery, G. K. (1983). Uncommon tiredness among college undergraduates. *Journal of Counseling and Clinical Psychology, 51,* 517-525.

Morris, M. L. (1982). Tiredness and fatigue. In C. Norris, *Concept clarification in nursing* (pp. 263-276). Rockville, MD: Aspen.

Morse, J. M. (1995). Exploring the theoretical basis of nursing using advanced techniques of concept analysis. *Advances in Nursing Science, 17*(3), 31-46.

Morse, J. M., & Carter, B. J. (1996). The essence of enduring and the expression of suffering: The reformulation of self. *Scholarly Inquiry for Nursing Practice, 10*(1), 43-60.

Morse, J. M., & Doberneck, B. M. (1995). Delineating the concept of hope. *IMAGE: Journal of Nursing Scholarship, 27,* 277-285.

Morse, J. M., Solberg, S., Neander, W., Bottorff, J., & Johnson, J. (1990). Concepts of caring and caring as a concept. *Advances in Nursing Science, 13,* 1-14.

Norris, C. M. (Ed.). (1982). *Concept clarification in nursing.* Rockville, MD: Aspen.

Patton, M. Q. (1980). *Qualitative evaluation methods.* Beverly Hills, CA: Sage.

Pugh, L. C. (1990). Psychophysiological correlates of fatigue during childbirth. *Dissertation Abstracts International, 51,* 01-B.

Pugh, L., & Milligan, R. (1993). A framework for the study of childbearing fatigue. *Advances in Nursing Science, 15,* 60-70.

Putt, A. (1975). Effects of noise on fatigue in healthy middle-aged adults. *Communicating Nursing Research, 8,* 24-40.

Radloff, L.S. (1977). The CES-D scale: A self-report depression scale for research in the general population. *Applied Psychological Measurement, 1*(3), 385-401.

Rhoten, D. (1982). Fatigue and the postsurgical patient. In C. Norris (Ed.), *Concept clarification in nursing* (pp. 277-300). Rockville, MD: Aspen.

Robson, K. M. (1982, June 9). An anxious time. *Nursing Mirror*, 15-17.

Walker, L. O., & Avant, K. C. (1995). *Strategies for theory construction in nursing.* (3rd ed.). Norwalk, CT: Appleton-Century-Crofts.

Waltz, C. F., Strickland, O. L., & Lenz, E. R. (1991). *Measurement in nursing research.* (2nd ed.). Philadelphia: F. A. Davis.

Wilson, J. (1969). *Thinking with concepts.* Cambridge, England: Cambridge University Press. (Original work published in 1963)

Yoshitake, H. (1971). Relations between the symptoms and the feeling of fatigue. *Ergonomics, 14*(1), 175-186.

Yoshitake, H. (1978). Three characteristic patterns of subjective fatigue symptoms. *Ergonomics, 21*, 231-233.

6

Development of a Conceptual Model of Quality of Life

Carol Estwing Ferrans, PhD, RN, FAAN

Quality of life (QOL) has become a critically important concept for health care in recent years. Quality of life considerations are significant in decisions to stop life-sustaining treatment and in debates regarding physician-assisted suicide. In clinical practice and clinical trials, QOL indicators are used to evaluate treatment in terms of human costs and benefits. QOL has also been used to make decisions regarding allocation of health care services, such as in Oregon's new health care system which has been viewed as a potential model for the nation. In this system, anticipated QOL outcomes were used to decide which treatments would be provided and denied to Oregon's poor (Hadorn, 1991). In addition, QOL has been proposed as a criterion for evaluating the quality of health care in a permanent national medical data base accessible to patients, payers, and providers (Elwood, 1988).

The literature reveals a wide variety of meanings for quality of life, defined explicitly or operationally (Ferrans, 1990a, 1992). Conceptual clarity is extremely important, because differences in meaning can lead to profound differences in outcomes for research, clinical practice, and allocation of health care resources. Concept analysis techniques using Wilson-based methods, predominantly those of Walker and Avant (1988), have been applied to QOL to help provide clarity (Kleinpell, 1991; Meeberg, 1993; Oleson, 1990b). A multiplicity of meanings can be identified from the literature using these techniques. The task breaks down, however, at the step of determining defining attributes. Because many definitions are mutually exclusive in their conceptual approach, they cannot be synthesized into a coherent whole. Hupcey and her colleagues (chapter 1) pointed out that Wilson-based approaches have produced results that lack cohesion and explanatory power. Morse and colleagues (chapter 4) then suggest that other approaches to concept analysis, such as critical analysis of the literature, qualitative methodologies, and quantitative methodologies may produce results that are more comprehensive and useful to nursing. Our work over the past 14 years in QOL provides an example of concept development using a variety of approaches. In addition to critical literature analysis and qualitative methodologies, we found that quantitative approaches can contribute meaningful information to concept development. Using these methodologies we developed a conceptual model of quality of life (Figure 6.1 and Table 6.1). This model provided the basis for the development of an instrument to measure QOL, which was our ultimate goal in this effort. The purpose of this chapter is to describe this work.

IDEOLOGICAL APPROACH

We began the work of explicating the concept of quality of life for instrument development in 1982. The first step was to select the ideological approach that was most appropriate for our purpose. We chose the individualistic view, in which individuals personally define what quality of life is for them (Edlund & Tancredi, 1985). Campbell, Converse, and Rodgers (1976) have argued that the essence of quality of life lies in the experience of life. The person is the only proper judge of his or her experience (Calman, 1987; Ferrans & Powers, 1985b; Neugarten, Havinghurst, & Tobin, 1961). The individualistic approach recognizes that different people value different things. Because of this, there is no single quality of life for all people with the same life condition (Hastings Center, 1987). A condition that makes life not worth living for one person may be only a nuisance to another. Early evidence of this was presented by Flanagan (1982), who found variation among the

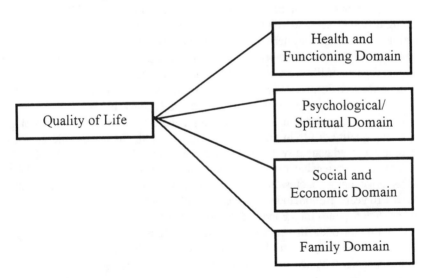

Figure 6.1. Ferrans's (1990b) Conceptual model for quality of life.

TABLE 6.1 Elements of the Ferrans Conceptual Model for Quality of Life

Health and Functioning Domain	*Social and Economic Domain*
Usefulness to others	Standard of living
Physical independence	Financial independence
Ability to meet family responsibilities	Home (house, apartment)
Own health	Neighborhood
Pain	Job/Unemployment
Energy (fatigue)	Friends
Stress or worries	Emotional support from others
Control over own life	Education
Leisure time activities	
Potential for a happy old age/retirement	*Family Domain*
Ability to travel on vacations	Family happiness
Potential for a long life	Children
Sex life	Relationship with spouse
Health care	Family health

Psychological/Spiritual Domain
Satisfaction with life
Happiness in general
Satisfaction with self
Achievement of personal goals
Peace of mind
Personal appearance
Faith in God

general population in importance of various aspects of quality of life, particularly among different age and gender groups. We also found evidence of this in our qualitative study of long-term survivors of cancer regarding their mastectomies (Ferrans, 1994) and in a number of studies that asked patients to rate how important various aspects of life were to them (Arzouman, Dudas, Ferrans, & Holm, 1991; Bihl, Ferrans, & Powers, 1988; Bliley & Ferrans, 1993; Ferrans, Cohen, & Smith, 1992; Ferrans & Powers, 1993; Hicks, Larson, & Ferrans, 1992).

When we began explicating the concept, there was no dominant ideology regarding quality of life in the literature. Since then, the individualistic view has become accepted generally. Evidence of this was provided by Osoba (1994), who performed an extensive literature search of MEDLINE and CANCERLIT to characterize major conclusions that could be drawn from quality of life research in the past 10 years. He concluded that quality of life is defined as a subjective concept, and as such depends on the individual's perspective.

Examination of the literature revealed six major conceptualizations of quality of life: the ability to live a normal life, ability to live a socially useful life (social utility), natural capacity (physical and mental capabilities), achievement of personal goals, happiness/affect, and satisfaction with life (Ferrans, 1987, 1990a, 1992). Of these, conceptualizing quality of life in terms of satisfaction was most congruent with the individualistic approach. The ability to live a normal life, a socially useful life, or have various natural capacities does not necessarily require a personal evaluation of the experience of life and may not be valued by the individual. Goal achievement itself also may not be valued by the individual. The notion of achievement of personal goals reflects the self-actualization ideals of Maslow (Edlund & Tancredi, 1985) and so may not be meaningful to all cultural groups. In contrast, happiness is universally meaningful, and discussion of this universal nature is found as early as Aristotle's *Nicomachean Ethics*. Current use of the term happiness, however, implies a transitory feeling or mood, whereas satisfaction implies a long-term judgment of life's conditions; satisfaction is thus more suitable for conceptualization of quality of life (Campbell et al., 1976). Satisfaction was also chosen because it implies a cognitive experience resulting from judgment of life's conditions (Campbell et al., 1976). As such, it fits well with an individualistic ideology. In addition, our definition focuses on satisfaction with the areas of life that are important to the individual. By this, the values of the individual are explicitly taken into consideration. Adhering to an individualistic ideology, we defined quality of life as "a person's sense of well-being that stems from satisfaction or dissatisfaction with the areas of life that are important to him/her" (Ferrans, 1985, p. 6; Ferrans, 1990b, p. 15).

ELEMENTS OF QUALITY OF LIFE

The second step in explicating quality of life was to determine the domain of content. A three-part approach was used. First, we used qualitative methodology to elicit from patients what quality of life was for them, which was congruent with the individualistic ideology we had chosen (Ferrans, 1982; Ferrans & Powers, 1985a). We interviewed 40 hemodialysis patients to determine the components of a satisfying life. Patients were asked to characterize the best and worst possible lives they could imagine in open-ended questions. Data were coded in terms of elements of life that were mentioned using inductive coding techniques (Glaser & Strauss, 1967). Twenty-two aspects of life were identified through the discussion of the best possible life, and 18 were identified through the worst. These findings were compared with other studies that asked the same questions of hemodialysis patients, arthritis patients, cardiac patients, kidney transplant patients, and the general population in 13 countries, including the United States (Cantril, 1965; Kilpatrick & Cantril, 1960; Hatz & Powers, 1980; Jackle, 1974; Laborde & Powers, 1980; Penckhofer & Holm, 1984; Sophie & Powers, 1979; Watts, 1981; Webb & Powers, 1982).

Second, we performed an extensive review of the literature from 1965 to 1983 through MEDLINE, CINAHL, and *Psychological Abstracts*. *Psychological Abstracts* alone listed 400 studies assessing life satisfaction for that period. Based on this literature review, a list of dimensions used in representative studies to assess quality of life was developed and published (Ferrans & Powers, 1985b). The data from our original qualitative analysis and from the literature review were synthe-sized to produce a listing of 32 elements of quality of life for the general population. Three additional elements were identified for dialysis patients (Ferrans & Powers, 1985b).

These elements were used as the basis for item development of the Ferrans and Powers Quality of Life Index (QLI). Each element was used to develop two items: one to assess satisfaction with the element and the other to assess its importance to the individual. The set of satisfaction items formed the first part of the instrument, and the set of importance items formed the second. Scoring was developed such that each satisfaction item was weighted by its paired importance item. This produced the highest scores for combinations of high satisfaction and high importance, and the lowest for low satisfaction and high importance. Weighting with low impor-tance produced middle-range scores. The rationale for the weighting scheme was the belief that people who are highly satisfied with areas of life they value enjoy a better quality of life than those who are dissatisfied with the areas of life they value. Thus, the quality of life score reflected satisfaction with the elements of life that mattered most to the individual, and so reflected the definition of quality of life that we had developed (Ferrans & Powers, 1985b).

The idea of measuring the importance of various elements has received support in the literature. In their critical appraisal of quality of life instruments, Gill and Feinstein (1994) argued that "quality of life may not be properly characterized unless patients are also invited to rate the importance of the problems" (p. 621). Support for this statement was provided by the findings of Blalock and associates (1992), who found that psychological well-being was impacted more by satisfac-tion with abilities than by the actual state of the abilities themselves. Further, they found that the influence of satisfaction with particular abilities was dependent on the importance placed on those abilities by the individuals in their study ($n = 234$).

DOMAINS OF QUALITY OF LIFE

The third task in concept explication was to cluster related elements together into domains of quality of life. We chose not to impose this structure based on our own reasoning, which would be inconsistent with the individualistic ideology we had adopted. Instead, we used exploratory factor analysis to determine the nature and number of the domains on the basis of patient data using the QLI. Factor analysis was performed on data from 349 hemodialysis patients who were randomly drawn from the hemodialysis patient population of Illinois (Ferrans & Powers, 1992). The maximum likelihood method was used for factor extraction, and the promax method for factor rotation. The number of factors was based on uniform results of five factor analytic criteria. The results revealed that four factors fit the data best, which represented the four interrelated domains of quality of life: health and functioning, psychological/spiritual, social and economic, and family. Higher order factor analysis performed on the factors demonstrated that the overall construct reflected in the entire set of elements was life satisfaction (Ferrans & Powers, 1992).

It is important to note that factor analysis produced results that were different from the conceptual structure we would have imposed. For example, we would have placed satisfaction with sex life together with satisfaction with spouse/significant other, thinking that both were related to marital life. These two aspects of life, however, loaded on different factors. Satisfaction with sex life was related to the health and functioning domain, and satisfaction with spouse was related to the family domain. These findings made conceptual sense in that they demonstrated that sex life was viewed as a component of health-related functioning, and that relationships with spouses entailed much more than sex life. Dialysis patients commonly experience sexual dysfunction related to renal failure (Berkman, Katz, & Weissman, 1982). This does not translate simply into dissatisfaction with their spouses, however. Even when patients have experienced loss of their sex lives, they have reported that they receive a great deal of support from their spouses and find satisfaction in their relationships with them (Berkman et al., 1982; Johnson, McCauley, & Copley, 1982; Murphy, 1982).

External validation of our conceptual model has been provided by the work of Ferrell, Padilla, Grant and their colleagues (Ferrell, Dow, Leigh, Ly, & Gulasekaram, 1995; Ferrell et al., 1992; Ferrell, Grant, & Padilla, 1991; Ferrell, Wisdom, & Wenzl, 1989; Grant et al., 1992; Padilla, Ferrell, Grant, & Rhiner, 1990). They also developed a conceptual model of quality of life based on qualitative analysis of data from patients, in this case cancer patients. The four components of quality of life in their model are physical well-being and symptoms, social well-being, psychological well-being, and spiritual well-being (Ferrell, Dow, Leigh, Ly, & Gulasekaram, 1995; Ferrell, Wisdom, & Wenzl, 1989). The close match between their model and ours provides mutual validation of the two models in that they were developed independently and simultaneously on the basis of patient data primarily from different sections of the country (i.e., the West Coast and the Midwest).

Additional support for the model can be drawn from the literature in that our model is consistent with prevailing views regarding the domains of quality of life. Table 6.2 presents summaries of the literature that have characterized the domains of QOL. These domains are remarkably similar to each other and to our model. One domain that is included in our model but is not in Table 6.1 is the family domain. It may be that other authors have nested it within the social domain. There is support in the literature, however, for family life as a crucial component of quality of life (Goodinson & Singleton, 1989; Jalowiec, 1990; Jassak & Knafl, 1990). In a representative U. S. sample, family life explained 28% of the variance in quality of life, which exceeded that explained by health or standard of living (Campbell et al., 1976). Adults with chronic illnesses ($n = 227$) also have identified family relationships as an important area of quality of life (Burckhardt, Woods, Schultz, & Ziebarth, 1989).

EXTENSION TO OTHER CULTURAL GROUPS

Our purpose in concept explication was to develop a measure of quality of life. The instrument we developed was the Ferrans and Powers Quality of Life Index, which was shown to be reliable and valid across a number of patient groups (Bliley & Ferrans, 1993; Cowan, Young-Graham, & Cochrane, 1992; Ferrans, 1990b; Ferrans & Powers, 1985b; Ferrans & Powers, 1992; Hicks, Larson, & Ferrans, 1992; Hughes, 1993; Oleson, 1990b; Papadantonaki, Stotts, & Paul, 1994). The patient populations used to develop the conceptual model and instrument, however, were predominantly middle- to upper-class Whites. Because of this, we wondered whether the conceptual framework appropriately reflected the thoughts and feelings of individuals from other segments of the population. To develop a measure of quality of life valid for other cultural groups, we needed to determine whether our conceptualization of quality of life was *etic*, or whether changes would be needed to reflect culturally specific elements. *Etic* concepts are truly universal across multiple cultural groups. *Emic* concepts have meaning only within a specific cultural or socioeconomic group (Triandis & Marin, 1983).

Specifically, we wished to develop measures of quality of life that would be valid for African Americans and Mexican Americans with low education levels. To accomplish this, it was necessary to validate our original conceptual model in these groups. For the Mexican Americans we simultaneously needed to establish linguistic appropriateness in Mexican Spanish.

We began by conducting three focus groups with African Americans: one with male cancer patients and two with female cancer patients. The results of these groups were consistent with the conceptual model, and we were reassured of the validity of the four domains for these patients. Next, all of the elements of the original model were examined using cognitive interview techniques. The methodology was based on cognitive research on the validity of responses to survey questions (Strack & Martin, 1987; Tourangeau, 1987; Tourangeau & Rasinski, 1988). During the interviews respondents were encouraged to "think aloud" about the thought processes used to respond to the question. Cognitive probes were designed to explore understanding of the various aspects of quality of life, how respondents retrieved information and formed judgments regarding the importance of and their satisfaction with each element, and whether they edited their responses. Question revisions were made iteratively, and each element was tested until responses became redundant (Warnecke et al., 1996).

Twenty-three African American and 15 Mexican American cancer patients were interviewed. The Mexican Americans spoke Spanish only or had Spanish as their primary language. Spanish was the primary language for the interviewers of the Mexican Americans. Of the elements of quality of life in the original model, only two were found to be *emic*. One was the ability to travel on vacations. The concept of vacation was meaningless for many respondents. If they traveled, it was for a family visit or emergency. This element was dropped when it became clear that the idea of traveling for pleasure had no relevance to their experience or life-style (Warnecke et al., 1996).

TABLE 6.2 Domains of Quality of Life from Summaries of the Literature

George & Bearon 1980	Spilker 1990	Osoba 1994
• Health and functioning	• Physical	• Physical
• Self-esteem	• Psychological	• Emotional
• Life satisfaction		• Cognitive
• Socioeconomic	• Social	• Social
	• Economic	

The second *emic* aspect of life was the idea of standard of living. Both the African American and Mexican American respondents had difficulty with this notion. Some interpreted it as addressing moral standards for living. In addition, there was no straightforward translation of the concept into Spanish. The element was dropped after efforts were unsuccessful at producing a consistent understanding of meaning. Other economic aspects of the model were relevant to respondents, however, such as financial needs, job, home, and neighborhood (Warnecke et al., 1996).

In summary, two of the elements of the original conceptual model were found to be irrelevant for the African American and Mexican American respondents. Interpretive problems were found for 11 elements, but they were appropriately reworded, and the interviews demonstrated that they were relevant in their reworded form. For example, "leisure time activities" was reworded as "things you do for fun." "Physical independence" was reworded as "ability to take care of yourself without help. " The 11 reworded elements and all the remaining elements were found to be universal across the two cultural groups for these respondents (Warnecke et al., 1996). Currently, we are continuing to test these elements with larger numbers of subjects in both groups using quantitative methodology.

An additional important finding was that the *emic* elements were found primarily through interviews with respondents who spoke Spanish only. Those who were bilingual were able to think in both English and Spanish, and so had linguistic access to the dominant American culture as well as Mexican American culture. The importance of this finding lies in the fact that the current gold standard for translation is Brislin's translation and back-translation approach (Brislin, 1970, 1986), which is performed by bilingual translators. These findings demonstrate that this approach cannot be depended on to achieve cultural appropriateness. Another step is needed with respondents who are monolingual to validly identify whether elements are culturally specific or universal (Warnecke et al., 1996).

CONCLUSION

In contrast to other concepts, quality of life was not adopted into nursing as a well-developed concept from another discipline. Instead, quality of life has been developed as a multidisciplinary effort over the past three decades. Nurses have made important contributions that have shaped the construct, and our work is one example of this. In this work we have not used a Wilson-based approach for concept development, but rather used qualitative methodologies for the initial identification of the elements of quality of life and for the development of the concept for other cultural groups. In addition, factor analysis provided a means to cluster elements on the basis of patient data. Thus, qualitative and quantitative techniques provided the methodologies for us to explicate the concept in a manner that was consistent with the individualistic ideology that we adopted. We also used literature review to provide insight into the responses of other samples and populations beyond those accessible to us. Based on these approaches, we developed a conceptual model that identifies four domains of quality of life: health and functioning, social and economic, psychological/spiritual, and family.

External validation of this model has been provided by its consistency with the work of others within and outside of nursing. The utility of the conceptual model has been demonstrated by its use as a framework by researchers in their publications and research studies. In addition, it provided the basis for development of the Ferrans and Powers Quality of Life Index. This instrument is being used in research and clinical practice in 18 countries by nurses, physicians, psychologists, and other professionals, and has been translated into 9 languages. Through its use as a framework for research and a basis for the instrument, the conceptual model has contributed to a better understanding of the impact of illness and treatment on quality of life.

REFERENCES

Aristotle. (trans. 1947). Ethica nicomachea. In R. McKeon (Ed.), *Introduction to Aristotle* (pp. 308-331). New York: Modern Library.

Arzouman, J., Dudas, S., Ferrans, C., & Holm, K. (1991). Quality of life of patients with sarcoma postchemotherapy. *Oncology Nursing Forum, 18*, 889-894.

Berkman, A., Katz, L., & Weissman, R. (1982). Sexuality and the life-style of home dialysis patients. *Archives of Physical Medicine and Rehabilitation, 63*, 272-275.

Bihl, M., Ferrans, C., & Powers, M. (1988). Comparison of stressors and quality of life of CAPD and hemodialysis patients. *American Nephrology Nurses Association Journal, 15*, 27-37.

Blalock, S., DeVellis, B., DeVellis, R., Giorgino, K., Sauter, S., Jordan, J., Keefe, F., & Mutran, E. (1992). Psychological well-being among people with recently diagnosed rheumatoid arthritis. *Arthritis and Rheumatism, 35*, 1267-1272.

Bliley, A., & Ferrans, C. (1993). Quality of life after coronary angioplasty. *Heart & Lung, 22*(3), 193-199.

Brislin, R. (1970). Back-translation for cross-cultural research. *Journal of Cross-Cultural Psychology, 1*, 185-216.

Brislin, R. (1986). The wording and translation of research instruments. In W. Lonner & J. Berry (Eds.), *Field methods in cross-cultural research* (pp. 137-164). Beverly Hills, CA: Sage.

Burckhardt, C., Woods, S., Schultz, A., & Ziebarth, D. (1989). Quality of life of adults with chronic illness: A psychometric study. *Research in Nursing & Health, 12*, 347-354.

Calman, K. (1987). Definitions and dimensions of quality of life. In N. K. Aaronson & J. Beckman (Eds.), *The quality of life of cancer patients* (pp. 1-9). New York: Raven Press.

Campbell, A., Converse, P., & Rogers, W. (1976). *The quality of American life.* New York: Russell Sage Foundation.

Cantril, H. (1965). *The patterns of human concerns.* New Brunswick, NJ: Rutgers University Press.

Cowan, M., Young-Graham, K., & Cochrane, B. (1992). Comparison of a theory of quality of life between myocardial infarction and malignant melanoma: A pilot study. *Progress in Cardiovascular Nursing, 7,* 18-28.

Edlund, M., & Tancredi, L. (1985). Quality of life: An ideological critique. *Perspectives in Biology and Medicine, 28,* 591-607.

Elwood, P. (1988). Shattuck lecture—Outcomes management: A technology of patient experience. *New England Journal of Medicine, 318,* 1549-1556.

Ferrans, C. E. (1982). *Factors influencing hemodialysis patient return to work.* Master's thesis, University of Illinois, Chicago, IL.

Ferrans, C. E. (1985). *Psychometric assessment of a quality of life index.* Doctoral dissertation. University of Illinois, Chicago, IL.

Ferrans, C. E. (1987). Hemodialysis: Quality of life as a criterion for allocation of life-sustaining treatment. In G. Anderson & V. Glesnes-Anderson (Eds.), *Health care ethics: A guide for decision makers* (pp. 109-124). Rockville, MD: Aspen Systems Corporation.

Ferrans, C. E. (1990a). Quality of life: Conceptual issues. *Seminars in Oncology Nursing, 6*(4), 248-254.

Ferrans, C. E. (1990b). Development of a quality of life index for patients with cancer. *Oncology Nursing Forum, 17*(3) *suppl,* 15-19.

Ferrans, C. E. (1992). Conceptualizations of quality of life in cardiovascular research. *Progress in Cardiovascular Nursing, 7*(1), 2-6.

Ferrans, C. E. (1994). Quality of life through the eyes of survivors of breast cancer. *Oncology Nursing Forum, 21*(10), 1645-1651.

Ferrans, C. E., Cohen, F., & Smith, K. (1992). Quality of life of persons with narcolepsy. *Grief, Loss, and Care, 5,* 23-32.

Ferrans, C. E., & Powers, M. (1985a). Employment potential of hemodialysis patients. *Nursing Research, 34,* 273-277.

Ferrans, C. E., & Powers, M. (1985b). Quality of Life Index: Development and psychometric properties. *Advances in Nursing Science, 8,* 15-24.

Ferrans, C. E., & Powers, M. (1992). Psychometric assessment of the Quality of Life Index. *Research in Nursing and Health, 15,* 29-38.

Ferrans, C. E., & Powers, M. (1993). Quality of life of hemodialysis patients. *American Nephrology Nurses Association Journal, 20*(5), 575-581.

Ferrell, B., Dow, K., Leigh, S., Ly, J., & Gulasekaram, P. (1995). Quality of life in long-term cancer survivors. *Oncology Nursing Forum, 22*(6), 915-922.

Ferrell, B., Grant, M., & Padilla, G. (1991). Experience of pain and perceptions of quality of life: Validation of a conceptual model. *Hospice Journal, 7*(3), 9-24.

Ferrell, B., Grant, M., Schmidt, G., Rhiner, M., Whitehead, C., Fonbuena, P., & Forman, S. (1992). The meaning of quality of life for bone marrow transplant survivors. Part I: The impact of bone marrow transplant on QOL. *Cancer Nursing, 15,* 153-160.

Ferrell, B., Wisdom, C., & Wenzl, C. (1989). QOL as an outcome variable in the management of cancer pain. *Cancer, 63,* 2321-2327.

Flanagan, J. (1982). Measurement of quality of life: Current state of the art. *Archives of Physical Medicine and Rehabilitation, 63,* 56-59.

George, L., & Bearon, L. (1980). *Quality of life in older persons.* New York: Human Sciences Press.

Gill, T., & Feinstein, A. (1994). A critical appraisal of the quality of quality-of-life measurements. *Journal of the American Medical Association, 272*(8), 619-626.

Glaser, B., & Strauss, A. (1967). *The discovery of grounded theory: Strategies for qualitative research.* Chicago: Aldine.

Goodinson, S., & Singleton, B. (1989). Quality of life: A critical review of current concepts, measures, and their clinical implications. *International Journal of Nursing Studies, 26,* 327-341.

Grant, M., Ferrell, B., Schmidt, G., Fonbuena, P., Niland, J., & Forman, S. (1992). Measurement of quality of life in bone marrow transplantation survivors. *Quality of Life Research, 1,* 375-384.

Hadorn, D. (1991). The Oregon priority-setting exercise: Quality of life and public policy. *Hastings Center Report, 21,* 11-16.

Hastings Center. (1987). *Guidelines on the termination of life-sustaining treatment and the care of the dying.* Bloomington, IN: Indiana University Press.

Hatz, P., & Powers, M. (1980). Factors related to satisfaction with life for patients on hemodialysis. *Journal of the American Association of Nephrology Nurses and Technicians, 1,* 290-295.

Hicks, F., Larson, J., & Ferrans, C. (1992). Quality of life after liver transplant. *Research in Nursing and Health, 15,* 111-119.

Hughes, K. K. (1993). Psychosocial and functional status of breast cancer patients. *Cancer Nursing, 16*(3), 222-229.

Hupcey, J., Morse, J., Lenz, E., & Tasón, M. (1996). Wilsonian methods of concept analysis: A critique. *Scholarly Inquiry for Nursing Practice, 10*(3), 185-210.

Jackle, M. (1974). Life satisfaction and kidney dialysis. *Nursing Forum, 13,* 360-370.

Jalowiec, A. (1990). Issues in using multiple measures of quality of life. *Seminars in Oncology Nursing, 6,* 271-277.

Jassak, P., & Knafl, K. (1990). Quality of family life: Exploration of a concept. *Seminars in Oncology Nursing, 6,* 298-308.

Johnson, J., McCauley, C., & Copley, J. (1982). The quality of life of hemodialysis and transplant patients. *Kidney International, 22,* 286-291.

Kilpatrick, F., & Cantril, H. (1960). Self-anchoring scaling: A measure of individual's unique reality worlds. *Journal of Individual Psychology, 16,* 158-170.

Kleinpell, R. (1991). Concept analysis of quality of life. *Dimensions of Critical Care Nursing, 10*(4), 223-229.

Laborde, J., & Powers, M. (1980). Satisfaction with life for patients undergoing hemodialysis and patients suffering from osteoarthritis. *Research in Nursing and Health, 3,* 19-23.

Meeberg, G. (1993). Quality of life: A concept analysis. *Journal of Advanced Nursing, 18,* 32-38.

Morse, J. M., Hupcey, J., Mitcham, C., & Lenz, E. (1996). Concept analysis in nursing research: A critical appraisal. *Scholarly Inquiry for Nursing Practice, 10*(3), 253-277.

Murphy, S. (1982). *Factors influencing adjustment and quality of life of hemodialysis patients: A multivariate approach.* Unpublished doctoral dissertation, University of Illinois, Chicago, IL.

Neugarten, G., Havinghurst, R., & Tobin, R. (1961). The measure of life satisfaction. *Journal of Gerontology, 16,* 134-143.

Oleson, M. (1990a). Content validity of the Quality of Life Index. *Applied Nursing Research, 3*(3), 126-127.

Oleson, M. (1990b). Subjectively perceived quality of life. *Image: Journal of Nursing Scholarship, 22*(3), 187-190.

Osoba, D. (1994). Lessons learned from measuring health-related quality of life in oncology. *Journal of Clinical Oncology, 12*(3), 608-616.

Padilla, G., Ferrell, B., Grant, M., & Rhiner, M. (1990). Defining the content domain of quality of life for cancer patients with pain. *Cancer Nursing, 13,* 108-115.

Papadantonaki, A., Stotts, N., & Paul, S. (1994). Comparison of quality of life before and after coronary artery bypass surgery and percutaneous transluminal angioplasty. *Heart and Lung, 23*(1), 45-52.

Penckofer, S., & Holm, K. (1984). Early appraisal of coronary revascularization on quality of life. *Nursing Research, 33,* 60-63.

Sophie, L., & Powers, M. (1979). Life satisfaction and social function: Post-transplant self-evaluation. *Dialysis and Transplantation, 8,* 1198-1202.

Spilker, B. (1990). Introduction. In B. Spilker (Ed.), *Quality of life assessments in clinical trials* (pp. 3-9). New York: Raven.

Strack, F., & Martin, L. L. (1987). Thinking, judging, and communicating: A process account of context effects in attitude surveys. In H. J. Hippler, N. Schwarz, & S. Sudman (Eds.), *Social information processing and survey methodology* (pp. 123-148). New York: Springer-Verlag.

Strauss, A., & Corbin, J. (1990). *Basics of qualitative research: Grounded theory procedures and techniques.* Newbury Park, CA: Sage.

Tourangeau, R. (1987). Attitude measurement: A cognitive perspective. In H. J. Hippler, N. Schwarz, & S. Sudman (Eds.), *Social information processing and survey methodology* (pp. 149-162). New York: Springer-Verlag.

Tourangeau, R., & Rasinski, K. A. (1988). Cognitive processes underlying context effects in attitude measurement. *Psychological Bulletin, 103,* 209-314.

Triandis, H., & Marin, G. (1983). Etic plus emic versus pseudoetic: A test of a basic assumption of contemporary cross-cultural psychology. *Journal of Cross-Cultural Psychology, 14,* 489-500.

Walker, C., & Avant, K. (1988). *Strategies for theory construction in nursing* (3rd ed.). Norwalk, CT: Appleton-Century-Crofts.

Warnecke, R., Ferrans, C., Johnson, T., Chapa-Resendez, G., O'Rourke, D., Chavez, N., Dudas, S., Smith, E., Martinez-Schallmoser, L., Hand, R., & Lad, T. (1996). Measuring quality of life in culturally diverse populations. *Journal of the National Cancer Institute Monographs, 20,* 29-38.

Watts, W. (1981). The future can fend for itself. *Psychology Today, 15,* 36-48.

Webb, S., & Powers, M. (1982). Evaluation of life satisfaction and sexual function in female patients postrenal transplant. *Dialysis and Transplantation, 11,* 799-804.

Index

Springer Publishing Company

Selected Writings of Rosemary Ellis
In Search of the Meaning of Nursing Science

Joyce Fitzpatrick, PhD, RN and **Ida Martinson,** PhD, RN

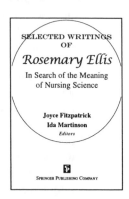

SELECTED WRITINGS
OF
Rosemary Ellis
In Search of the Meaning
of Nursing Science

Joyce Fitzpatrick
Ida Martinson
Editors

SPRINGER PUBLISHING COMPANY

Dr. Rosemary Ellis (1919-1986) was one of nursing's most penetrating thinkers and treasured scholars. Here, for the first time, is a collection of many previously unpublished writings as well as several of her classic publications. In these writings, Dr. Ellis tries to get to the very essence of nursing science, and to lay the philosophical groundwork for the development of theory and research to improve nursing practice. Written with unusual clarity of thought and expression, nurse researchers, theorists, educators, and graduate students will find this a fundamental resource.

Contents:

- Explanatory Knowledge for Nursing: Forms and Approaches
- Characteristics of Significant Theories
- Values and Vicissitudes — The Scientist Nurse
- Training for Research
- Humans as Instruments of Science
- Philosophic Inquiry
- Knowledge for Nursing Practice
- Nursing Knowledge Development
- Theory Development in Nursing: The State of the Art
- Nursing Scholarship and Nursing Practice
- Nursing Research: Diversity in Scientific Inquiry

1996   152pp   0-8261-9400-1   hardcover

536 Broadway, New York, NY 10012-3955 • (212) 431-4370 • Fax (212) 941-7842

℗ *Springer Publishing Company*

Annual Review of
Nursing Research, Volume 15

Joyce J. Fitzpatrick, PhD
Jane Norbeck, DNSc, Editors

Now in its second decade of publication, this landmark series draws together and critically reviews all the existing research in specific areas of nursing practice, nursing care delivery, nursing education, and the professional aspects of nursing.

Contents:

1997   340pp (est.)   0-8261-8234-8   *hardcover*

536 Broadway, New York, NY 10012-3955 • (212) 431-4370 • Fax (212) 941-7842

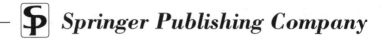

Springer Publishing Company

Using the Arts and Humanities to Teach Nursing
A Creative Approach

Theresa M. Valiga, EdD, RN
Elizabeth R. Bruderle, MSN, RN

This is a comprehensive sourcebook on using the humanities to teach nursing concepts. The authors, who have used the humanities to teach nursing at Villanova's College of Nursing since 1985, first give a general introduction to literature, television, film, and fine arts along with advantages and disadvantages of using each in nursing. They then describe selected nursing concepts, and provide specific examples of works of art that can be used to illustrate each.

> SPRINGER SERIES ON
> TEACHING OF NURSING
>
> **Using the Arts and Humanities to Teach Nursing**
> A Creative Approach
>
> THERESA M. VALIGA
> ELIZABETH R. BRUDERLE
>
> This comprehensive sourcebook is designed to help nurse educators be more creative in their teaching by using the humanities. The authors explain how the teaching of nursing, may benefit from integrating elements of literature, television, film, and fine arts. The authors then describe selected nursing concepts along with specific examples of works of art that can be used to illustrate each concept.
> The numerous artworks discussed in the book include novels, short stories, children's literature, poetry, films, television, music, sculpture, paintings, opera, photography, and drama.
> This book can be used by faculty in any nursing education program—graduate, baccalaureate, associate degree, diploma, or LPN—and by staff development educators as well.
>
> SPRINGER PUBLISHING COMPANY

These works include a variety of art forms — novels, short stories, children's literature, poetry, films, television, music, sculpture, paintings, opera, photography, and drama. The book is designed so that nurse educators can integrate this material into standard nursing courses, and it can be used by the faculty in graduate, baccalaureate, associate degree, diploma, LPN, or staff development education.

Springer Series on The Teaching of Nursing
1996   320pp   0-8261-9420-6   hardcover

536 Broadway, New York, NY 10012-3955 • (212) 431-4370 • Fax (212) 941-7842